The Decoded Sh*t For Life

crack the code to achieve

success & happiness You desire

Alayna Sonar

Published by

Copyright © <Alayna Sonar > 2023

All Rights Reserved.

ISBN 978-93-90994-09-0

Book is about:

<u>After reading the book- Realization:</u>

Sahinahihai wo loghai jo kehtahai "Sabko sab kuchnahimilta." "ItnaAasaannahihaiZindagiJeena". "Life is always too hard to understand" "Its too difficult to live in this world". Let me tell you a truth my friend

"Rules are Rules & Brulés are Brulé". Humme se bahut log Brules (so called laws made by the society) ko life rules samajh ka apnizindagi me aagenaibadh pate) In a world filled with negative messages and limiting beliefs, it can be easy to get distracted or disheartened. For example – Shaddi ki umarhotihai, log kyasochega, duniya wale kyabolenga……

This book offers a New Perspective, one that acknowledges the power of the mind includes magic to overcome even the most deeply ingrained patterns of thinking and behavior. Above are not the universal law which can't be changed, We as a Human are much powerful with the power of our Mind and to be specific Sub-conscious mind, and the programming which has done in our mind since we were born is a myth* which we have to REIMPRINT our SUB_CONCIOUS MIND with the Formulas and break your unworthy pattern and live a life of FULFILLMENT.

"Pyaar, Paisa aur Power – sab mileage wo bhisath me" if You feel that Your Dreamer is Still Alive and agree to WORK/CHANGE/IMPROVE your action then GO FOR IT and implement NOW the learning from this book. It's so simple to live a *life of Abundance, Happiness, Success, Love And all that You ever dream of.*

Note: Brulés - Also known as "bullshit rules," are unwritten cultural norms or expectations that people are expected to follow. These norms are often deeply ingrained in society and may not align with our personal values or beliefs. – You have the Rights to break such Brulés

The Decoded Sh*t

For Life

A book of Contagious happiness & Success in LIFE

"The Decoded Sh*t for Life" by Alayna is an insightful and transformative self-help book that offers readers a new approach to achieving success and happiness in every aspect of life. With practical advice, personal anecdotes, and a healthy dose of humor, Alayna provides readers with the components they need to decode the challenges of life and create a life they love.

Through her candid and relatable writing style, Alayna tackles a wide range of topics, from overcoming fear and self-doubt to achieving career success and building strong relationships. Drawing on her own experiences and the wisdom of others, she offers practical advice and actionable steps that readers can take to start making positive changes in their lives today.

"The Decoded Sh*t of Life" is a refreshing and empowering guide to living your best life. Whether you're just starting out on your journey or looking to make significant changes, Alayna's book will inspire you to take action and create a life that is truly fulfilling and meaningful. With her straight-talking, no-nonsense approach, Alayna cuts through the noise and offers readers a roadmap to success that is both practical and achievable.

Let's Make A DEAL

Choose wisely MONEY/TIME

With The value of 10$ or 1000RS what you can Purchase? and what's the value of 20 Min in YOUR Life? Can you calculate what you can get in exchange for your money? You surely can get anything that's equal to that value, right?

But one thing for sure you can't buy with infinite money exchange and that's "The precious TIME of Your LIFE. TIME waits for none... It's my genuine recommendation. Please choose wisely where you actually get the maximum benefits out of it. This book is one handy manual for all your answers. Read it to get the maximum benefits and save your precious time. (Tag me Your thoughts @my Instagram handle @alayna_sonar before reading this book>>> valuable thoughts would love to read your experiences in this Format –

(Before & After Effects) You can find the difference in Your perspective

Let me remind you 1 thing – Perception is Projection

NAME - ____

County/Region - ___________________________________

Book purchase date - ______________________________

What's going Thoughts inside you BEFORE reading this book -

____

Pen down your Thoughts AFTER Reading this Book -

____

I Devoted my entire life to studying and researching, Helping people around the world in these areas of concern, and then bundled up the most inestimable information (Treasure)t into a neat little package to share with the world.

Books Are The Most Undervalued Commodity On The Planet

Earn some Extra Money / Lose some extra FAT, wanted to do something and actually doing it, are two totally different ball games. We are all busy with our Jobs/Business, our Family / Friends, our kids (IF we have :) plus we have to get some beauty sleep, household chaos, Walk or jog, and of course, we have to find the time for some Netflix/dramas, chill & party (Apology if your stuff is not in list but the list goes on and on) Now a days social media contents are so addictive that we keep on scrolling, but we hardly use our time in our self-growth, self-love and the end story lies the same, the whole day just went off in the blink of eyes.

If you Value TIME & MONEY BOTH

then Choose to Read THIS BOOK

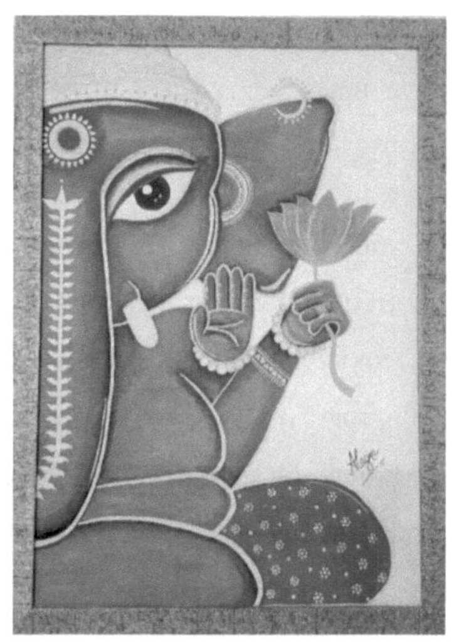

I'M BLESSED

GANPATI BAPPA MORYA

THE DECODED SH*T FOR LIFE:

"UNLOCK YOUR POTENTIAL: THE ULTIMATE GUIDE TO LEARNING AND GROWING" IS A TRANSFORMATIVE SELF-HELP BOOK THAT OFFERS READERS A POWERFUL FRAMEWORK FOR UNLOCKING THEIR FULL POTENTIAL AND ACHIEVING

THEIR LIFE GOALS. WITH A FOCUS ON EXPLORING NEW IDEAS AND EXPANDING YOUR KNOWLEDGE, THIS BOOK OFFERS A FRESH PERSPECTIVE ON PERSONAL GROWTH AND LEARNING.

IN A WORLD WHERE INFORMATION IS EVERYWHERE, IT CAN BE OVERWHELMING TO KNOW WHERE TO START. THAT'S WHERE "UNLOCK YOUR POTENTIAL" COMES IN. WITH A WEALTH OF NEW AND GAME-CHANGING IDEAS, THIS BOOK OFFERS A ROADMAP FOR EXPLORING THE NEAR-INFINITE MASS OF INFORMATION AVAILABLE TO US, AND FINDING THE IDEAS AND CONCEPTS THAT ARE MOST RELEVANT TO OUR LIVES AND GOALS.

THROUGH A COMBINATION OF PRACTICAL ADVICE AND INSPIRING STORIES, "UNLOCK YOUR POTENTIAL" SHOWS READERS HOW TO REFRAME THEIR MINDSET, EMBRACE NEW IDEAS, AND DEVELOP THE SKILLS AND HABITS NEEDED TO SUCCEED IN ANY ENDEAVOR. WHETHER YOU'RE LOOKING FOR ADVANCE IN YOUR CAREER, IMPROVE YOUR RELATIONSHIPS, OR SIMPLY BECOME A MORE KNOWLEDGEABLE AND WELL-ROUNDED PERSON, THIS BOOK IS A MUST-READ FOR ANYONE LOOKING TO UNLOCK THEIR FULL POTENTIAL AND ACHIEVE THEIR DREAMS BY THESE SIMPLE LESSONS

ENDNOTES

GOOD VIBES GOOD LIFE - VEX KING

THE SHIT THEY NEVER TAUGHT YOU_-_ADAM JONES & ADAM ASHTON

THANKYOU

CONTENTS

<u>Personal Information</u>

I grew up in a loving family of four who lived a simple and comfortable life in our own way in a middle-class community. Although we faced our fair share of struggles, my family always taught me the value of appreciating the small things in life and finding fulfillment in them. My father was especially instrumental in instilling these values in us.As an average student, I completed my graduation and started working at a small firm. However, I didn't let that stop me from pursuing my dreams further education and enhancing my skills. I went on to study for an MBA along with job, determined to improve myself and reach my full potential and explore the world.

After spending 12 years in various prestigious MNC firm in India, I began to feel hollow and unfulfilled. Despite earning good and providing a good lifestyle for my family, I felt lost and unsure of my purpose of my being. The loss of my beloved father only made matters worse, leaving me even more distraught.

For a while, I continued the same path as working 9-6 sometimes even moreworking extensively. I was just doing for the living but my soul was hungry for something else, I married the love of my life that I decided to take a step back and search for the purpose of my life. As my both families supported in my decision and with everything settled in my personal life, I felt the freedom to pursue my calling. I left my job and embarked on a journey of self-discovery. Although I continue to fulfill my responsibilities to my family, I am now doing so with renewed purpose and clarity.

Earlier I was living in a messy state. I felt detached from the world, I felt like I had closed all the doors and windows to breathe, and I was just working aimlessly without any direction. I was constantly feeling sad, depressed, and argumentative with others, In a state of "victimhood,"

I believed that everyone else was responsible for my life except me. With no clear purpose, I felt suffocated. I searched for answers from experienced people but never found the solution. As I was a workaholic person but after leaving the job my world was surrounded with only few people that was the best part but, I love to be a social person, involve self in various activities, helping people around, but felt more isolated and incomplete from inside. Society thinks that as You get married to a good family what else do you need, but deep inside me a war was going on for what I don't know, I was restless and yearned for meaning in my life.

I read the weather report that "Tonight there will he Meteor shower I was very much exited to see it, I love stars, Visiting Northern light is my dream, On that dark and cold night, as I sat sipping hot tea on the terrace with a warm fire beside me and stars above, the thought hit me hard even more that I was living a worthless life, without direction or purpose. It was a turning point that made me start a journey towards evolving myself limitlessly. Today, I can confidently say that I have all the ingredients required to be called as a HAPPY SOUL, & a successful person as per societybrules. In the modern world: I am happy, wealthy, loved, smart, and competent in all areas of life, people do love me and admire me as who I am. I love being around people, I love to explore the World.

The journey wasn't easy, but I learned that the key is to trust the process and to carry your confidence with you. The little things that I learned along the way were surprisingly simple, but no one had ever taught them to me before. You must have faith in your journey, even if it seems like nothing is happening. Just like a bamboo tree that takes years to show any signs of growth, but then suddenly blooms into the tallest tree in the forest within months.

Life is like a forest, and to make your presence felt, you must deepen your skills and work on yourself a little more every day. But first, you have to find your place in this world, your reason for being. This book is a manual for a happy life, filled with tiny chapters that will guide you towards self-growth, self-love, self-worth, success, and happiness. It's not a magic pill, but it will become an addiction for those seeking to better themselves.

I feel blessed to be able to share these insights with others, to simplify the process of living a beautiful and precious life, just like in the movie "Zindagi Na Milegi Dobara". This book is a reminder that success and happiness are within reach for anyone who is willing to put in the heart and trust the journey.

Throughout the book, you're going to hear out from me –

Through deep introspection and research, I have discovered my true self and become the best version of ME. Armed with this new found knowledge, I am now committed to contributing to society bysharing my experiences and knowledge, helping others to achieve the life they desire.

My personal journey has taught me the importance of self-awareness, self-care, and pursuing one's passions. By sharing my story and the lessons I have learned, I hope to inspire and empower others to discover their own path to fulfilment and happiness.

Whether it is through mentorship, public speaking, or simply being a positive role model, I am dedicated to making a difference in the lives of those around me. I firmly believe that by helping others with these courses live their best lives, we can all create a better, more compassionate world.

"Depth of Beginning" Signatureprogram - Synergy Transformation Journey

"Evolve Limitless"One of the most loved courses for Life & Mind& Magic

"Astonishing You"Master yourself with the Power hidden inside YOU

"DIVA-Wings" Only for the Divas - A life transformation Journey of

Finding self and Gaining POWER Back

<u>Disclaimer</u>

I believe that this book contains valuable life lessons that can help readers achieve their desired state from their current state, provided they are willing to learn and apply the lessons in their life. It is an exclusive book as it is the first ever written in my line of ancestors, and I feel a sense of responsibility to share the golden words that can bring a positive revolution in the heart and mind of the reader. However, I also acknowledge that there are many factors that contribute to a person's current state, and while my book can certainly help individuals improve their circumstances, it is not a magic solution that will immediately solve all problems. Ultimately, it is up to the reader to determine how they want to approach the lessons and apply them to their life.

I've designed this book to be concise and to the point, catering to those who may not have a lot of free time or a strong passion for reading but still desire to gain knowledge and develop new skills. My goal is to transform the lives of people who are determined to become respected members of society, bring about positive change, and achieve success in their lives by sharing life-changing lessons that were not taught in traditional educational institutions. By incorporating my personal life experiences into the book, I hope to provide readers with valuable insight and avoid repeating the same mistakes that I made in my own journey.

As an avid reader myself, I strongly believe in the power of books to enhance knowledge and understanding, ultimately serving as a timesaving and life-saving resource. I've intentionally avoided using fancy language or unnecessary fluff to ensure that the content remains accessible and practical for all readers.

The content of this book will be Crisp and clear Codes and Decodes of Life. So let's start as if you are starting a New Journey to become **"Astonishing You"**

My inspiring mission to bring joy and happiness into the lives of others and make a profound and positive impact on the world.

When thinking about life, Remember these Lines :

No Amount of <u>Guilt</u> can change your <u>Past</u>

No Amount of <u>Anxiety</u> can change your <u>Future</u>

Life can only be <u>Understood backwards</u>

But it <u>SHOULD</u> be <u>Lived Forward</u>...

Dedicate

I devote this book with lots of love in the memory of

My Beloved Father - Late Shri Dindayal Sonar Ji

You will always be my hero and my first love. *As all daughters share this lovable bond with their Father*, My Dadaa words of encouragement have been a constant source of strength and motivation for me throughout my life. He taught me an invaluable lesson during our upbringing - to never consider us weak or inferior because We were girls. He always referred to me as his strong pillar, and his words have left a deep impression on my heart. Heartfelt Gratitude to his encouragement here I'm.

He modeled honesty, integrity, and hard work in everything he did, and I learned from him the importance of living a life based on these values. He taught me that success is not just about achieving material wealth or status, but about living a life of purpose and meaning. He always reminded me to be grateful for the blessings in my life and to never take anything for granted. He taught me to appreciate the simple pleasures of life, such as spending time with family and friends, and to always be kind and compassionate towards others.

His love and guidance have been the driving force behind my success, and I am forever grateful for his unwavering support. Though he is no longer with me, his memory lives on, and I carry his lessons and love with me every day. Dad, your daughter will always be your shining star. I love you and miss you deeply, and "I dedicate this book to you as a testament to the impact you had on my life."

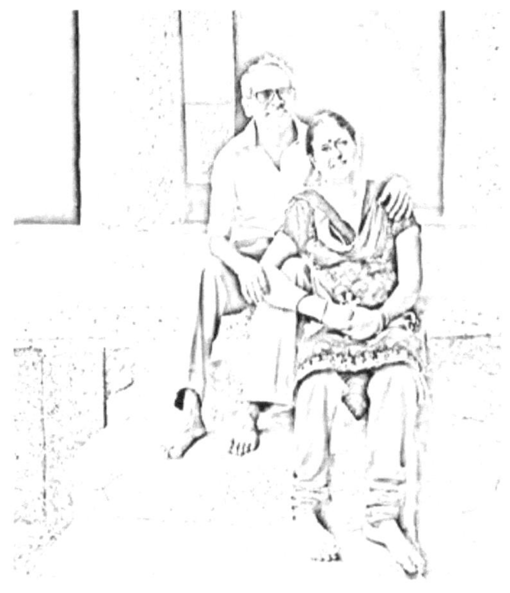

<u>Dadda & Maa</u>

Maa...

The living inspiration of my life, Meri Maa, I dedicate this book with all my heart. Our life has been challenging, but your unwavering strength, faith, and perseverance have made incredible things happen for us. Your sacrifices, determination, and endless love have been the foundation of my life, and I am forever grateful for all that you have done. You are an inspiration to me, and your guidance has been invaluable on my journey. I hope this book honors your unwavering commitment to our family and the tremendous impact you've had on my life. Maa, I love you, and I dedicate this book to you with immense gratitude and admiration."

<u>Acknowledge</u>

Suneel, my beloved partner, and closest confidant, you have shown me nothing but unconditional love and support, even in the face of adversity and my own mistakes. Your love has been the driving force behind the sacrifices you've made for me, and it is your love that has kept me going and given me the strength to pursue my dreams. You have forgiven me, hugged me, laughed with me, inspired me, encouraged me, and healed me, demonstrating that with love, anything is possible. Your selflessness has inspired me to follow in your footsteps, and through my words, I hope to spread that same love and positivity to others.

Mummy Papa I feel incredibly blessed to have such wonderful in-laws, who have always treated me like their own daughter and supported me in being true to myself, even if it meant going against societal norms. I can't express how much their love and acceptance means to me, and I'm forever grateful for the endless power they've given me to pursue my dreams and live life on my own terms. Much needed love and support continue to inspire me

To my gorgeous sister*Pratima*(Piya) I want you to know that you are more than just a sibling to me - you are my cherished first daughter, my trusted advisor, & my dearest friend. Your presence in my life has been a constant source of comfort & joy, Your love and unwavering support have been invaluable to me, Our bond is truly magical, & the moments we share together are some of the most precious memories I hold dear. I am grateful for the countless ways you have been my partner in crime, through thick and thin, Thank You for being a constant light in my life, and for bringing so much warmth and love into our family

Part I

Connection for Happiness

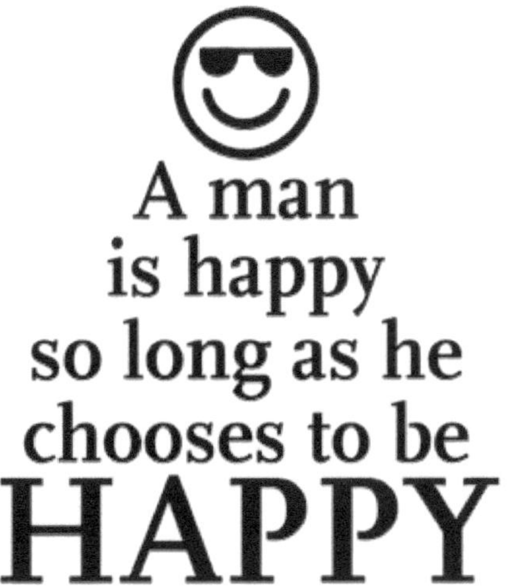

Sh*t no 1

<u>Magical Point in Life:</u>

The thought we all have is that if we do all of the right things now, then at some MAGICAL POINT in the future we will be happy.

Is it so Guys?

I Believe this prevalent idea is that if we follow all the right steps and make the right choices in the present, then we will eventually reach a point in the future where we will be magically happy. However, this notion is flawed somewhere because it places too much emphasis on external factors and future outcomes, rather than on the present moment and our internal state of being.

Happiness is not a destination that can be reached by simply ticking off a list of accomplishments or achieving certain external goals. Instead, true happiness comes from within and is a product of our mindset, perspective, and daily habits. It is essential that we focus on cultivating a positive and grateful mindset, living in the present moment, and nurturing positive relationships and experiences in our daily lives.

Many of us find ourselves stuck in a cycle between step one and step two, endlessly pursuing new achievements without ever reaching step three, which is essential for experiencing true fulfillment. We might put in extra hours at work to earn a promotion, only to find ourselves continuously striving for the next promotion. Or we may focus on learning new skills to land a good job, but then feel compelled to keep acquiring more knowledge without ever feeling satisfied. We might even achieve significant success, only to immediately move onto the next project without ever taking a moment to appreciate our accomplishments. It seems like happiness is always just out of reach.

It's important to reflect on whether we are truly caught in this cycle forever or if we can break free from it. We must ask ourselves if we are currently experiencing genuine happiness and satisfaction, or if we are merely pursuing external achievements without finding true fulfillment. While continuing to learn and grow is important, we need to take time to appreciate our accomplishments and savor the moments of happiness and contentment that arise along the way. By being mindful of our goals and taking time to appreciate our achievements, we can break free from the cycle and experience greater happiness and satisfaction in our lives.

If we trudge (walk slowly and with heavy steps) through the mud and the slime, if we get battered and bruised (hurt) by the storm, then once the sun comes out the other side, we'll find our pot of gold at the end of the rainbow.

In simple words

The common belief is that if we persist through difficulties and challenges, even if we have to trudge through mud and slime or endure the battering of storms, we will eventually reach a point where we find our pot of gold at the end of the rainbow.

While it's important to persevere through challenges and not give up at the first sign of difficulty, it's also crucial to recognize that there is no guarantee of reward waiting for us at the end of the journey. Life is unpredictable, and even our best efforts may not always lead to the outcome we desire.

Humneaksar kai bar sunahaibado se, apne parents, grand parents se ki beta/betiabimannlaga k padh lo aagezidagi bahut khubsurathojayegi... (*Hogi –future tense)*

In our 10th,12th Graduation or any other dam courses/syllabus which we get enroll forcefully sometimes, Fir jab hum wo karletahai to fir JOB/CAREER/BUSINESS me 18-35 age me hum khud ko samjhatehai, log boltehaiabimehnatkar le jawan hai experience le lo sikhojitna mile aur hum apna pura bachpan aur jawaniisibhag-daud meinbhuladetahai ki abikar le bad me enjoy karega ...

Ye jhoot ki "Poori life padi (*left*)hai enjoy karne k liye" iss beech Shadi aur Bachaabhi ho jatehai(*contition apply**) Hume patabhinaichalta ki hum ek phase se dusre phase me kab jump kardetahai.. Fir hum apnese chote ko b wahi same story samjhatehai.. and the cycle goes on and on from generation to generation.

Most people think the path to success looks like this:

Study Hard* > *Work Hard* > *Enjoy Happiness

Work Overtime* > *Get Promoted* > *Be Happy

Great Work* > *Great Success* > *Great Happiness

However, this model is flawed.

Between step one and step two, we are stuck in a loop that never ends, preventing us from reaching step three, which is crucial.

We work extra hours to get a promotion, but instead of being satisfied, we just keep working extra hours to get the next promotion. To get a good job, we learn new skills, but instead of being happy, we keep learning new skills. We put in a lot of effort, get a big success, and then immediately get back to work on the next project. Happiness never arrives. When you can continue your education and earn a master's degree, why stop at a college degree? When you can work harder and become a Vice President, why stop at Director? When you could continue working and saving for a second investment property, why settle for just one? Happiness always goes further and further away from us. Just want to ask you guys: Are you really looped in this chain forever? Can you ask Yourself, that the moment of your happiness and feeling of satisfaction is still alive in you now?

IF not then Try to be *Happy at theMoment* in which ever you have at presentTHE MAGICAL POINT IS NOW TO BE HAPPY

Fortunately, there is an easy fix.

Simply change the equation around:

Be Happy First. Here's what your new path should look like:

Be Happy ↠ Great Work ↠ Big Success

Happy people are 31% more productive, 37% more likely to sell there products and services, and three times more creative than unhappy According to Harvard Business Review. People who are happier perform better at work and advance in their careers.They are happier in their relationships and at home. Therefore, we ought to all just smile constantly.

Its Ezzzyyyyyy (easy) to say BE HAPPY But we know that it's not quite that simple in reality. That's because our perception of 'happiness' is out of whack.Happiness does not mean the absence of negative thoughts. We all havenegative thoughts! There is no such thing as an eternal optimist – negativeself-talk always creeps in. So the problem is not that we have negativethoughts in our brain - the problem is that we think we shouldn't havenegative thoughts.If you're seeking out trouble to solve, you're going to find a problem.Instead of always looking for what is wrong with our life, why don't wefocus on what is right and what we can change?

Be happy first ⬤ *This will definitely change your perception*

Zindagidekhne ka nazariyabadalkedekho,

Zindaginabadletohkehna...

A Poem:

Kitne sawal kitne veham kitni uljhane

Mann mein liye chalte rahoge...

kitni bar mutthiyon se ret ka fisalna ka

wo ehsaas liye chalte rahoge

 Wo Jo tumhara nahi hai uske milne ki

pyaas liye chalte rahoge...

Kitne ilzaam odhoge aur kitni bechainiyan

sametoge

Ek bar sar uthakar khud se najre milakar

dhundh lo vo rasta

Jo pighla dega tumhare pairon ki janzeer...

Wo rasta Jo tumhen Apne aksh se milvaega

usse Dosti karvaega

Jara Gaur se dekho wo rasta, Kahi yahi se

hokar gujarta hai

Shayad tumhare wajood ki tarah,

Use bai dhak liya hai kuchh pareshaniyon

ne...

Par Jara Gaur se dekho tumhare andar se

hokar guzarta hai wah raasta

Jahan Aasman aur jameen milte Hai, Aaj

iss pal milte hai...

Wo rasta tumhare hi intezar mein bichaa hai

Bus der hai To tumhare haan kahane ki

To chalo Aaj jindagi ko han kahate hai

To chalo Aaj har Khushi ko haan keh de

Jo bhi hai bas Yahi ek pal hai

---Anonyms

Dear soul,

You are the essence of my being, the very core of my existence. You are the part of me that remains constant through the ups and downs of life, the part that knows my true desires and aspirations.

You are the voice that guides me towards my true purpose, and the light that illuminates my path. It is true that we all have an ocean inside of us, a vast and infinite sea of emotions, thoughts, and feelings. Yet, so often we forget to dive deep within ourselves to explore this ocean, instead seeking outside sources to quench our thirst for knowledge and fulfillment.

But my dear soul, I vow to always remember the ocean within me, and to nurture it with love, curiosity, and a deep sense of connection to the world around me. I will listen to your whispers and follow your guidance, trusting that you will lead me to my highest potential and help me fulfill my purpose in this world.Thank you for being a part of me, dear soul. I promise to honour you always.

With love and gratitude, Your human self.

Sh*t no 2

Here we will do an exercise of our thoughts:There are 168 hours in a week. Divided time roughly in the boxes.

Let's fill the **1st** box with sleep/rest time i.e., 8hrs of sleep (8x7=56hrs), **2nd** with Work/Activities lets assume 10-12 hrs including travelling (12x7=84hrs) now This indicates that we still have the **3rd** box. This week, we have 28 hours to do whatever we want. Although 28 hours per week should be sufficient, you probably believe you require more. Sleeping and working, are precisely thethings we need to give us the time/energy/money/structure to do whateverwe want in bucket three. However, this equation varies from one individual to another. More or less we must have to take time for the 3rd BOX but most people squander (waste) Ignore the **SELF*ME*** TIME

Explaining with my life example:As an IT professional in a large service industry firm, my team and I had a very demanding workload. We were responsible for ensuring that the services provided by the company were operational 24/7. While some teams within the company seemed to have more leisure time, my team had to be constantly available to respond to any issues or upgrades required. This often meant working through the night to ensure that services were reactivated before the start of the business day.

It could be frustrating at times to see other teams seemingly enjoying more relaxed schedules while my team had to work tirelessly to keep everything running smoothly.

However, we were dedicated to our work and understood the importance of meeting deadlines and ensuring that services were always functioning properly.

If something went wrong on a Friday, we actually felt relieved because it meant we had two full days to work on the issue before the start of the new work week. On the other hand, if upgrades or changes were needed on a Friday, we had to sacrifice our weekends to ensure that everything was completed before Monday morning. It was a challenging job, but we were committed to delivering high-quality service to our customers.

No matter the field, work can be challenging and demanding, especially for those who spend long hours in the office and have to endure daily commutes. I share this example not to discourage you, but to help you understand that many people experience similar struggles and can relate to the pain and frustration that comes with hard work. However, it's important to maintain a positive mindset and find ways to prioritize self-care and balance, even amidst the demands of work. Remember, you are not alone in your challenges and there are ways to overcome them.

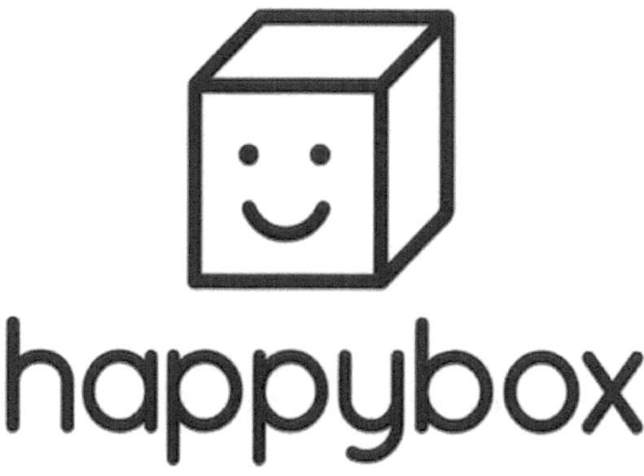

We are living in

"A BOX LIFE"

Ek box shape k bed se soke uthatehai, box room me fresh hotehai, tiffin Box me khana le jatehai, Box structure vehicle (car/train/bus..etc) me travel kar k office pahuchtahai, Box shape office building me enter kartehai, box lift, then reach to our box shape Desk or cabin, work on Box Laptop/desktop and during lunch box shape oven me khana garam kartehai aur pet bhartehai, fir sham ko box shape coffee/team machine se Chai/ coffee pitehai, fir box files ko review ya report banatehai, Box bag leka office se nikal k fir box vehicle me travel kar k Box ghar me jatehai aur fir wahi box bed me dinner kar k so jatehai… Most pity part is that thoda sab bhi time mile to, we involve ourself in BOX shape Cell Phones or TV (So called Smart Phone & Smart TV)these are really kills our smartness

It's important to set boundaries and limits on our technology use, and to prioritize activities that promote our overall well-being, such as physical activity, socializing with friends and family, and engaging in creative or meaningful pursuits.

Hope this made you realize that we are totally boxed in our life and we have no space to breath, kabhikabarbaharghumnechalegaye to baat hi kuch aur hai aur agar box resorts/restaurants/malls me naigaye to bahut achi baat hai..

So guys we are screwed up, all the activities which are required, complete your task & responsibility, BUT BUTBUT… also fill the 3 BOX with "The Happiness"

 Do all stuff that makes you happy and Alive, things you actually love to do, your hobbies, find your passion, spend time with your loved once, and self-love is most important as I have always said.

GOLDEN RULE: Many people ask me "mujhe to pata hi nahihaimujhekisme Khushi miltihai"… So I want to tell them ki apne life me kuchnaya explore kiya hi naihai bus jabsehoshsambhalawahikarteaayeho jo sabne kaha… Par abb wo karo jo apkokarnahai, but make sure your action should not hurt others. Explore new adventures in life.

Example : Make new friend, explore the world, try new dishes, new activities, new things aur jaisa hi aapkuchnayakarnashurukaroge you will find kuch to aisa that you really love to do and you will surely find Your kind of

Happiness…

Achieving happiness requires deliberate consideration of the path that is right for you. While some people may prioritize a job based solely on its yearly salary, it's important to also consider the hourly wage and the impact on other areas of your life. If your work commitments are starting to encroach on the time and energy you need for other things you enjoy, it's likely that your overall happiness will suffer. In such a situation, it's crucial to reassess your priorities and realign your life to ensure that you can enjoy a fulfilling and balanced existence.

Sh*t no 3

Say <u>STOP</u> to Worries & Stress

DON'T LET THE **PAST**(No longer Exist)

BLACKMAIL YOUR **PRESENT**(Gift)

TO RUIN YOUR BEAUTIFUL **FUTURE**(Unavailable now)

We have heard/read these statements many times, "Stop worrying about the past. Stop worrying about the future. Live in the present."

The child says: "When I am a big Girl ...". But the big girl says: "When I grow up...". Then the grown-up says: "When I start earning" When a financially independent girl says, "When I get married...". Then the married women say: "when my children are born, "The Mother says, "When my children's are grown up and settled" Then the mother inside you says "When I'm able to retire after my children's are married ..." Similarly goes with Men's as well. But when they retire and look back over their shoulder, somehow, he/she misses the roses they strolled past every day. Life is slipping away @ incredible speed. We are racing through space at a rate of 30 km/sec. Today is our most precious possession. It is our only sure possession.

(Waqtbaditezi se guzartahaijanaab, patabhinaichalta, aur jab mud kedekhtahai tab tak bahut der ho chukihotihai…

Nazarebadalte der nahilagti…)

Life is in Now (*ZindagiAaj ka naam hai*) but we learn this too late. The great French philosopher Montaigne quipped has quoted so beautifully:

"My life has been full of terrible misfortunes,

Most of which NEVER happened ".

We're so worried about what might go wrong thatwe miss all the things that go right. One of the most tragic things about human nature is our tendency to put off living what is in front of us. We are all dreaming of some magical Butterfly rose garden over the horizon instead of enjoying the roses blooming right outside our windows.

Be Decisive

When you are worried about something, ask two questions:

1. *What am I worrying about?*

2. *What can I do about it?*

Then make a decision.

Most people get caught on step 1. All they worry about is… what

they're worried about it! We must make that second vital step and determine what we can *do* about it.

There is immense value in making a decision, even if it is not perfect. If we do not decide, we move forward in crazy circles that lead us to a living hell. Most worries seem to disappear as soon as you reach a clear final decision. The rest falls away when you make a decision and turn it into action.

Once you've made up your mind based on the facts, go straight to step no 2. Don't stop to reconsider. Don't hesitate. Don't worry and track your steps no 2. Don't lose your self-doubt. Don't look back over your shoulder. Just decide and then do it.

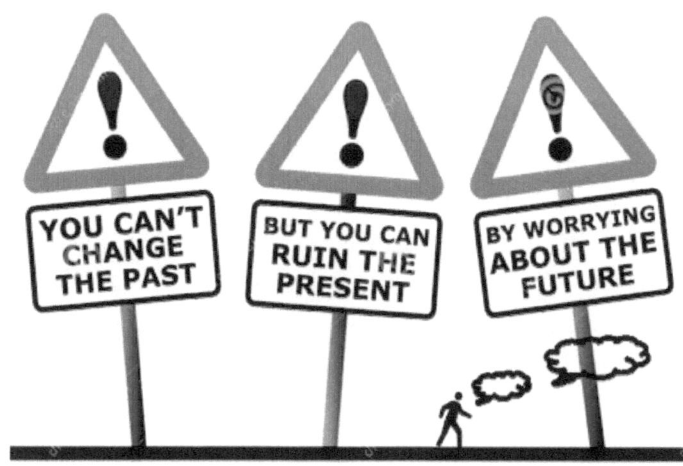

Sh*t no 4

Don't Expect Gratitude:

Shri Krishna ne kaha hai Karm karFal ki chinta mat kar.

(Though I don't believe it completely it varies from person to person or situation to situation) *You have to do your duty religiously and don't expect anything from anyone.*

Almost two thousand years ago, Marcus Aurelius wrote in his diary: *"I am going to meet people who talk too much, are selfish, egotistical, and ungrateful. I won't be surprised or disturbed, for I couldn't imagine a world without such people"*. Human nature has always been human nature. If BigMarcus was experiencing ungrateful people two millennia ago, what makesyou think people are going to change now? We can wish that the world was different, or we can be realistic and accept it for what it is. If we go around

grumbling about ingratitude, who is to blame? Is human nature at fault, or is it our ignorance of human nature?

Let's talk about our parents. Are we grateful for them every second of our life? What they did for us whole life, or is your child grateful for what you have sacrificed to give them a best life…

Let's not expect gratitude. If we don't get it, we won't be disturbed. But if we get it occasionally, it will come as a pleasant surprise. This point is also applicable for all the people around us

" A BIG ZERO EXPECTATION FROM ANYONE IS THE BEST MINDSET APPROACH "

Having zero expectations from others doesn't mean we shouldn't do anything for anyone or help them. It means that we should approach our actions with a selfless mindset and not expect anything in return. We should be kind and give the best we can from our whole heart without expecting any specific outcome or reward.

When we believe in the concept of karma, we understand that what we give out into the world will eventually come back to us in some form. This can be a powerful motivator to do good and be kind to others, without expecting anything in return. It can also help us let go of any attachments to outcomes and trust that what is meant for us will come our way.

In essence, having zero expectations and believing in karma can be powerful tools for cultivating a more selfless and fulfilling life, while also promoting kindness and compassion towards others.

The love of a mother is often described as something truly divine and magical. This unconditional love is a pure example of giving without expecting anything in return. Similarly, helping others without expecting anything in return can bring a sense of fulfillment and joy that is not dependent on external factors. In essence, true happiness comes from the act of giving and not from what we may receive in return.

Sh*t no 5

Quote by Dale Carnegie: "Nobody kicks a dead dog"

It is common for us to get caught up in negative emotions and self-sabotage, often as a result of external circumstances or the behavior of others. However, dwelling on these negative emotions and situations can be draining and ultimately serve no purpose.

One way to address this is to shift our focus and energy towards what does serve our well-being. This may involve letting go of situations or people that are no longer serving us or taking action to improve our own situation. It can also involve cultivating a more positive mindset and finding ways to focus on the good in our lives.

Rather than dwelling on negative emotions and self-sabotage, we can choose to shift our perspective and focus on what we can control and what serves our overall well-being. By doing so, we can avoid getting stuck in negative patterns and instead create a more positive and fulfilling life.

<u>Example:</u>If youLove someone with your whole heart can be a beautiful and fulfilling experience, but it can also bring a deep ache if that person is no longer in your life. This may be due to various reasons, such as death or a breakup, and the pain may feel overwhelming and difficult to heal.

However, it is possible to come out of that pain and move forward, even if the ache may never completely go away. One way to do this is to focus on living for the people who are still in your life and finding ways to cope with your emotions in a healthy way. This may involve seeking support from loved ones or a therapist, engaging in self-care activities, and finding new ways to bring joy and fulfillment into your life.

Although it may be difficult, it is important to remember that life is a gift and that we have the power to shape our own path. While the ache of losing someone we love may never fully go away, we can find ways to honor their memory and create a meaningful and fulfilling life for ourselves. In doing so, we not only honor the past but also create a brighter future for ourselves and those around us.

Jinhejanaatha wo chalegaye... Jo haiunkeliyesocho aur Jio...

Start living AGAIN

Making The Most of Bad Situations

One of the most remarkable characteristics of humans is their power to turn a minus into a plus. The most important thing in life is not to capitalize on your gains. Anyone can do that. The thing that will set you apart is your ability to profit from your losses. That requires intelligence. That's what separates the winners from the worriers. When life hands us a lemon, let'smake some lemonade. And when someone throws stone on you make a bridge out of it. The greatest gift of a human being is the Brain, and the capacity to think act accordingly. And you know one interesting thing we human have the ability to smile & express our emotions, is one of the unique characteristics of being human. A smile can be a powerful tool for changing our own mood and influencing the mood of those around us.

When we smile, it sends a message to our brain that we are happy, even if we are not feeling that way in the moment. This can trigger the release of endorphins, which are natural mood-boosters, and can help to lift our spirits and reduce stress levels. Additionally, when we smile, it can have a contagious effect on those around us. It can help to lighten the mood, ease tension, and promote a more positive atmosphere. This can be especially helpful in difficult or challenging situations, where a smile can help to shift the energy and create a more positive outcome.

So, bringing a smile to our face can be a powerful tool for turning a situation around and promoting a more positive outlook. Even in difficult times, a smile can help to lift our spirits and make us more resilient in the face of adversity.

Look On The Bright Side Always

"Our happiness depends on

the habit of mind we cultivate."

Inspired by: The Power of Positive Thinking,

by Norman Vincent Peale

Sh*t no 6

Good Vibes only:

The world in which you live is not determined by external conditions and circumstances, but by the thoughts that habitually occupy our minds. You can think your way to failure, or you can think your way to success.

William James, the Father of Psychology, said in the late 1800s: *"The greatest discovery of my generation is that human beings can alter their lives by altering the attitudes of mind .*

As you think, so shall you be".

Our thinking can take us to the top of the success ladder, or the pits of doom. As Henry Ford once said: *"If you think you can, You are Right, or If you think youcan't", you're probably right too"*. If you think you're a hopeless loser just here to hang around for a couple of decades without making any impact, then that is exactly what you will be. So flush out all your deep-rooted, drained, worn-out thoughts, and fill your mind with fresh, new inspired ones that will plant the seeds of a great life. Thinking is a big deal. Most people miss out on a good life due to their worthless thoughts. Thinking positively all day every day isn't the only ingredient for success, but thinking negatively is a sure path to failure and disaster.

Based on the Principle of LAW of Vibration, to receive good vibes we must project good vibes. The transmitter and receiver of vibration frequencies always pull in the same frequency just like a mirror. If I smile looking at the mirror the I in mirror smile back to me in the same frequency, instead of feeling good once you have it all, start feeling good from now. Truth is that if you want to become happy, act as if you are happy NOW with your wholehearted feeling as it's the only truth that you are happy now.

Ultimately the self-love and level of your vibration go hand in hand, by taking positive action and changing your thoughts you will manifestation greater things, It's a natures' law.

So, if you love and adore yourself you will live a life you love and adore the most.

Loving and adoring yourself is an important aspect of living a fulfilling and satisfying life. When we love and accept ourselves for who we are, we are more likely to make choices that are in line with our values and priorities. We are also more likely to attract positive experiences and relationships into our lives.

Self-love involves treating ourselves with kindness, compassion, and respect. It means prioritizing our own needs and taking care of our physical, emotional, and mental well-being. This may involve setting boundaries, practicing self-care, and being mindful of our thoughts and emotions.

When we love and adore ourselves, we are more likely to have a positive outlook on life and feel more confident in our abilities. This can lead to greater happiness, success, and fulfillment in all areas of our lives. By prioritizing our own well-being and self-love, we can create a life that we truly love and adore.

Take an Oath Right Now

I Choose Peace and Acceptance

I continue to become a Better Person Everyday

I know I can reach my Goals, So I am Committed to Achieve

them

I will ignore Negative Opinions on ME

I will Take care of my Body Physically & Mentally

I know That I deserve Great things in my Life

I'm Becoming Stronger & Unshakeable

I Surround Myself with Positive people

I'm happy and healthy, I'm loved and taken care of...

Just RELAX and LET GO
if it's meant to happen it will find a way.

FLOW with the UniverseFrequency

Embrace the Good Vibes, Learn to let it go with the flow Stop forcing yourself for Outcomes Aligned yourself in harmony with the Universe What is meant for You will surely find a path to come to you. When your heart is in something only good things can happen, Now that may not always be true, But always remember that Rejection are just redirections to the things which are far better for you, As we always heard "Jo hota hai ache ke liye hota hai" here I would like to add " Usme acha kya hai aap ko dhundna hai" Any failure you felt at that time is always a lesson to learn,

 Only with faith we can recognize the VALUE of our apparent downfall. What we truly want, often comes wrapped in different packaging!!!!!!!!!!!!!! Maybe

Aisa Bhi ho sakta hai a " Jo hum chahtehai wo kisi aur roop me humare pass aajaye"

Always learn to let go… And let things flow in their natural way… We should always try hard for what we desire to achieve but don't get stuck or obsessed with the outcome..

Let it go and be happy that your happiness lies somewhere else finding your happiness is the true journey of your life.

Rather I would like to say…

"BE happy and You will find your Happiness"

Sh*t no 7

<u>Make Yourself a Priority:</u>

Do remember always - That's not selfishness

You are never too selfish or weak to distance yourself from the crowd who always drains your energy, try to bring down your vibes, gossip or say ruthless things which make you uncomfortable.

The Life which you have received is a priceless gift and sharing it with the people who bring the best in you and love you unconditionally is the correct place for you to stay happy.

Prioritizing your own needs is not selfish. Sometimes, only you truly understand your own pain and circumstances, and it's important to take care of yourself.

For Example : If you order a small pizza that's meant to be shared among four people which suddenly appear, but you're hungry and ask for your fair share, others might view it as selfish. However, at that moment, you're simply prioritizing your own needs and there's nothing wrong with that. It's important to take care of yourself in order to lead a healthy and fulfilling life.

*Next time when
you think of
Beautiful things,
don't forget to
count yourself in.*

It's important to practice self-love and self-care, and to set aside time for yourself. While it's great to give love and energy to the world around us, we also need to take care of ourselves in order to maintain our own well-being. Practicing self-love and self-care can help us recharge and replenish our own energy, which in turn allows us to give even more to the world. It's important to prioritize and make time for activities that bring us joy and help us feel refreshed, whether that's meditation, exercise, reading, or simply spending time alone. By taking care of ourselves, we can lead more fulfilling & satisfying lives, & ultimately give even more to the world around us.

Yaad rakhna hamesha : Akela aayethay akela hi jayega, Par sabse gehra aur pyara Rishta apka, Apse hi hai..

If you can accomplish this relationship well with yourself, you surely can succeed with good relationships with others as well.

When we put ourselves last, we fall behind, Our dreams and goals become harder to find, But when we prioritize our own needs, We find the strength to plant new seeds.

Self-care isn't selfish, it's a necessity, To love ourselves is a divine responsibility, We can only give to others when we're fulfilled, So, prioritize yourself, it's the best gift to build.

In a world that demands so much of us, It's easy to lose ourselves in the fuss, But making yourself a priority is a must, To live a life that's full of trust.

So, my dear friend, make yourself a priority, Invest in your well-being with sincerity, You'll find the joy and peace you seek, When you realize your worth, and your power to speak.

In life's grand scheme, we often forget, To care for ourselves, our needs unmet, But like a flower that needs water and light, Our own well-being requires our sight.

When we prioritize our own self-care, We become stronger, more resilient, aware, We find the power to overcome and thrive, And tackle life's challenges with a drive.

So, my friend, make yourself a priority, Your mental and physical health a necessity, Take the time to nurture your mind and soul, And watch your life's happiness unfold.

Remember, you deserve love and care, So, be kind to yourself, always be aware, Your well-being matters, don't forget, Make yourself a priority, without regret.

Sh*t no 8

<u>Other side- Seems Always Bright:</u>

I have read somewhere these beautiful lines:

Flowers are Pretty but, So are Sunsets...

And they look nothing Alike...

Both are Beautiful in their way...

The Reason we are Struggling with Insecurity is Because

We are Compare our behind-the-scenes to everyone else's highlight reels...

---- Steve Furtick

Ek baat samaj lenajaisaapapnigaltiya aur failure chupate ho waisa hi log bhi chupati hai.. Hum wahidikanachahtehai jo acha hai khoobsurathai… to hum ye kyu nazar andaz kar jate hai ke log bhi aisa hi karte honge. Dusro ki Chakachaund me apni Roshni ko mat khona dena tum ek nayabheera ho bus der hai to dulha takne ki….

Don't compare Yourself...

You were born to be You.

Always Remember You are Unique..

By comparing! You are losing your Uniqueness..

Comparison is the most common reason why we experience sadness. I confess that comparison has stolen my joy on many occasions.

Here a little story from my life incident:

I remember during school I'd rarely invite my friends to my house because I felt embarrassed by its size and condition I was living in a Chawl, but now I feel that it was the most beautiful time of my life as all my childhood friend were always together near and never felt alone or sad always joyful surrounded with awesome people.

I still remember I was at the home alone my parents went outside for some work and I was playing (pakda pakdi) hope all remember, and I fall down and injured very badly, my knees were bleeding and ankle got twisted and it was unbearable pain literally speaking I felt like cry my eyes out of the extreme pain, and with in fraction of time crowd gathered and the neighboring aunties uncles took me to the hospital and I got plaster in my ankle and took care of all the hospital bliss as well though no one was so much financially capable of they contributed and whole day they took care of me and my younger sister who was just 3yrs not able to understand what's happening and was frightened but they all took good care of us, That day was a lavish buffet for us, all aunties bought varieties of food different cuisine like, Marathi, Bengali Punjabi Muslim aunty bought water bag, medicine, chocolates etc. Jisko jo samaj me aa raha tha was doing their best, I'm grateful and thankful for all of them for their whole life.

During those days cell phones were not available, so I was unable to contact my parents. They came late at night and saw everyone inside that little room. I felt much relief later after taking medicine and seeing Mumma papa thanks all of them . Now I felt that these were the greatest blessings in life, which most of us are missing nowadays.

Let's get back to the topic,

When we compare, we always look at those who we perceive to be doing better than us; rarely do we look at those who are facing bigger struggles than us. So we never feel grateful for what we do have.

Looking to others for inspiration

is OK , but there's a difference

between inspiration and envy.

Comparing our lives with others' that we see online is a waste of energy. People only share photos in which they look attractive, happy, and successful; not when they're tired, scared and lonely.

The rise of social media is proving problematic, too. Younger age groups of children and adults are now becoming heavily absorbed in it, unaware that social media presents rose-tinted versions of life as the truth, and it's against this fiction that they're comparing themselves. I've learned that sometimes real couples who are on the brink of giving up on their relationship will post a multitude of

loving images online so that no one realizes what they're going through and judges them. (Not that these couples would be likely to share their arguments and disagreements online instead; no one says halfway through an argument, 'Hold on, let me take a picture of this.') People will post remarks saluting how amazing the couple's relationship is and how they wish they could have the same thing – drawing a comparison. They have no idea what's happening behind the scenes.

Always Remember, if someone is sharing images or videos of their wonderful life, you don't know what they went through to get it. For every accomplishment, there might have been a bucket load of tears, blood and sweat. Even for some of the public figures who are constantly seen online as being in love, there might be a history of rejection and bullying. For every gorgeous photo, there may be 100' that were deleted back then.

It appeals to human nature to turn to social media for instant validation through likes, comments, and followers. When we engage with social media, our brain releases dopamine, a hormone that makes us feel good (and is also involved in addiction). Have you considered that you might be comparing your life with those of people who use social media to fill a void in themselves because they've forgotten how to practice self-love?

I've come across people who are completely different on social media than they are in real life. The truth is distorted with filters and inspirational captions to make everything seem better than it is. We all know this, but we fail to recall it. This isn't about what other people are doing or sharing online. It's not about what they're up to in life or how far they've gone. It's about you. *Your competition is you.* Give Your best in every/daily task, and that's where your comparison should be directed The person you were yesterday.

If you want to be the greatest version of yourself, you have to keep focus on your own life and goals. Improving 0.0001% everyday is also an Achievement of the better You.

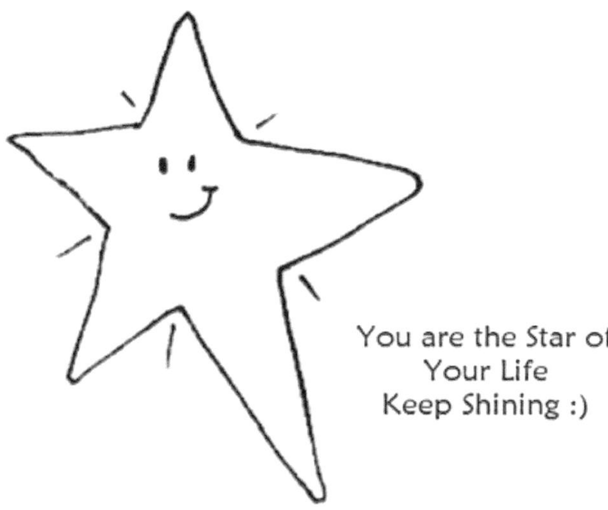

4 MANTRAS

TO HELP YOU STOP YOURSELF FROM COMPARING

NoBody is ME and That's MY SUPERPOWER

I give Myself Permission to Embrace All side of ME

I'm Grateful for Who ImE Who I'M becoming

I'M on the Path that is best for ME Right Now

Sh*t no 9

Money is form ofEnergy Exchange nothing more than that

Money flows like energy, free and pure, Neither good nor bad, a power to procure, In our Universe of infinite abundance and grace, A tool to assist, not a prize to chase.

Don't let wealth define or complete your soul, Rather, let it help you achieve your goal, Use its flow to create and spread joy, To empower yourself and others, and not destroy.With an open mind and heart, let money be, A means to support your dreams and set you free, For in this vast Universe, there's plenty to share, And with love as your guide, you'll always fare. Money is often viewed with different interpretations, some people believe that making money by pursuing their purpose is wrong. However, it is important to understand that money is not inherently good or bad, but simply a form of energy. The way we perceive and use money determines whether it brings positive or negative outcomes.

Money can be used to accomplish great things or it can reflect the misery that exists within the person's mind. In essence, money is an amplifier that magnifies the qualities of the person using it. Therefore, if one does not create value by spreading kindness and love when they have very little money, it is unlikely that they will do so when they have more of it.

The flow of money is often determined by the individual's beliefs and mindset. It is important to reflect on your views towards money & whether you believe that you deserve to have more of it.Your subconscious thoughts and feelings about money can have a significant impact on your current financial reality and your future experiences with money.

It is important to note that some people believe that money is the root of all evil, yet they still desire it. This contradictory mindset is similar to placing an order at a restaurant and walking out before having your meal. If you cancel your request for money, how can the Universe deliver it to you?

How can the Universe deliver a request you've already canceled? Some people feel guilty or ashamed for wanting more money because they are often labeled as greedy. However, the desire for financial freedom and the ability to live one's desired lifestyle without restriction is a common aspiration for many individuals.

For example, one might want to be able to take holidays with their loved ones without worrying about the cost. However, perceiving this desire as greed implies that the supply of money is limited and that others will never have the opportunity to break away from their current lifestyles to experience the same level of freedom.

In reality, money is abundant, and there is no limit to the amount of wealth that can be created. Furthermore, everyone has the potential to improve their financial situation and experience the freedom that comes with it. Therefore, there is no need to feel guilty for wanting financial abundance and living the lifestyle of your dreams.

Instead of thinking that there is a limited supply of what we want, we can reframe our mindset to believe that abundance is infinitely available and provided by the Universe. The Universe is abundant and constantly providing us with an endless supply of resources and opportunities. By embracing this perspective, we can open ourselves up to the infinite possibilities that exist and trust that the Universe will provide us with everything we need. With this abundance mindset, we can approach life with optimism and gratitude, knowing that we are surrounded by limitless potential for growth and fulfillment.

The Universe is abundant and always providing us with opportunities to prosper. However, our mindset plays a critical role in attracting abundance into our lives. When we focus on lack and limitation.

We emit a fear-based vibration that attracts more scarcity and difficulty. This can lead to a scarcity mentality where we become afraid to lose what we have and hold onto it tightly, creating further obstacles to financial abundance.

Rather than committing our energy to poverty, we should focus on prosperity and abundance. This does not mean we should spend recklessly or neglect our finances, but rather that we should approach money with a mindset of abundance and trust that we will always have enough. By shifting our focus towards prosperity, we can harness our creative power and attract wealth into our lives.

It is essential to recognize that money is not the sole source of happiness or purpose in life. We can add value to the world and serve others through our actions and contributions, regardless of our financial situation. Therefore, we must cultivate a mindset of abundance, not just for ourselves, but for the benefit of the collective consciousness. By doing so, we can empower ourselves and those around us to create a more prosperous and fulfilling world.

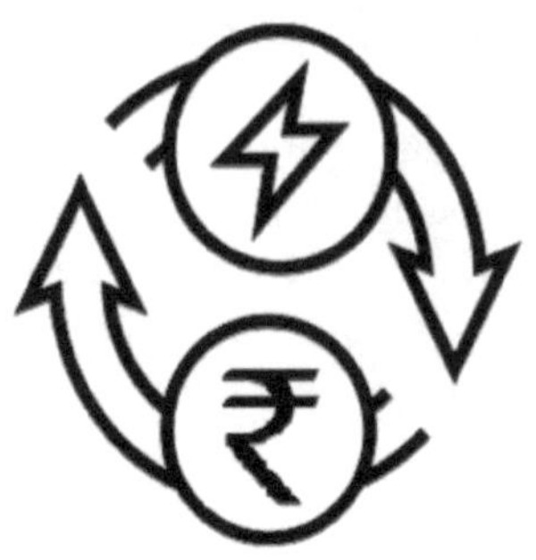

"Money is a form of energy, and it has its own unique vibration. When we align our energy with the vibration of money, we attract abundance into our lives."

- Denise Duffield-Thomas

Sh*t no 10

Let it Go Happiness comes from within

__You have to stop blaming yourself or others for the the miseries of your life

_Forgive Yourself

_For the Past Mistakes You have made

For the times you feel like You weren'tEnough

For the times You were in the Wrong

For the times You disappointed Yourself

For the Time You could have been more empathetic

For the Time You said things out of anger

For the lesson You learned a little too late

For the times you have realized

you were the Toxic one

For the time you didn't stand up for yourself

For the Time you didn't Trusting your instinct and made Wrong Decisions

And for the time being, not loving yourself Enough….

Very often We disrespect our own Individuality, our Existence and

intellect when we make a mistake!

 Do you ever ask yourself discouraging questions like, 'Why can't I do this?' 'Why am I so horrible?' or 'Why do I keep failing?' Why the hell does everything happen to me only? And more of such -ve statements …?

        Such an inner voice we have can be very dangerous. This type of question is often a presupposition, forcing you to accept the ideas in the questions as truth. It's a highly effective way to put yourself down. But you must make sure the voice in your head is always kind to you. You'll encounter many people in life who are willing to put you down, but *you* shouldn't be one of them.

YOUR BODY HEARS EVERYTHING YOUR MIND SAYS

You literally cannot expect others to be generous to you if you're not generous to yourself. You have to change your internal dialogue, so it supports you in life. Instead of telling yourself that you're dumb or an idiot making a mistake, tell yourself that you're only human and you'll do better next time for sure.

Your words are creative energy – an idea we'll expand on in the next section. They're extremely powerful in either supporting you or limiting your life experience. When you use words to belittle yourself, you diminish your own joy.

THE only REAL MISTAKE is the One From Which WE Learned NOTHING

- John .Powell

Do you still punish yourself for the mistakes you made as a teenager? IF the Answer is maybe NO, then it's too painful to carry that regret with you. And if it's a YES, that's because we realize that we were young and innocent, and most of us have learned from them. They've allowed us to become better. This self-forgiveness should apply to your recent mistakes, too. Every mistake you make can help you to improve as a person. But to make use of the lesson within each of your mistakes, you must first learn to let them go. Accept what has happened.

Anything that costs your peace is too Expensive…

Learn to BREATH SMILEY & Let it GO

Your SOUL Knows when it's TIME you Close the Chapter You're allowed to continue with life, regardless of the scale of the mistake (Big or Small). Don't punish yourself for what you've done, and instead focus on what you can do better. "TO heal a Wound, you need to Stop Touching it."

The truth is that 'You in the Past' was probably completely different from who you are now. So, if someone judges you for your past, it's their problem. They're the ones who are living in a place that no longer exists. If they don't understand that people grow up and mature, they probably have stuck in the past and created their own bubble.

Don't let anyone use your past as an excuse to judge you; they're only trying to restrict you from building a blissful future. Remember that nothing stays the same, includin

<u>Hear is a beautiful saying:</u>

Yesterday is a HISTORY

Tomorrow is MYSTERY

But Today is a GIFT...

That's why it's called PRESENT

PART II

SECRET ELEMENTS FOR MAGICAL TRANSFORMATION IN YOU

Sh*t no 11:

TRUE Purpose of LIFE

It did not really matter what we expected from life,

But rather what life expected from us.

— Victor Frankl

Life ultimately means taking responsibility and finding the right answer to problems that life assigns to each individual. Human life, under any circumstances, never ceases to have meaning.

The meaning of life is always changing :It is a bit like asking a chess master: "What is the best move in the world?" There is no such thing as the best or even an objectively 'good' move. There is only a specific 'good' move for each particular situation in each game against every particular opponent. Just as in life, each person has their own particular vocation or purpose to carry out at any given moment. Each situation in life represents a challenge and a problem to solve. Ultimately, we should not ask what the meaning of life is.

 Purpose isn't packeted up into tidy, perfect, Shiny moments,

Purpose may be born in sweat, tears, or hard days you went through

It may be born in the late dark lonely nights, hardest lesson or

Maybe you realize your Purpose in the most unknown territory or in the moments of happiness. I believe that everyone has a purpose in life: A purpose to be of service to the world. This purpose, along with the experience of unconditional love and joy, is the reason for our existence.

Purpose provides us with meaning to Life.

Most of us find it difficult to identify what our true purpose is.

Others have a feeling that they know what it is, but are often forced to imitate society's norms and reject their real purpose in the name of practicality.

Think of football. The purpose of this ball is to be kicked.

If the ball just sits there doing nothing in the corner of a room,

its purpose is being ignored – however, it doesn't care,because it has no soul. Imagine now that the ball has a soul,giving the ball self-awareness. If the ball stayed sitting in the corner of the room, it would have a strange feeling inside of it,like something was missing. The ball may never find fulfillment because it would probably feel as if it hasn't shown the world's true worth. He may be in comfort zone but unhappy

Now imagine someone finally picks up the ball and decides to throw it around. As the ball glides through the air, it feels ecstatic. But moments later, the ball feels a void inside itself again, because although it had fun, it wasn't enough.

The ball might then be used in a variety of ways, seeing plenty

of action but still feel unfulfilled. The ball assumes that the more events that occur in its life, the closer it'll come to fulfillment. But the more events it experiences, the more this idea is disproved.

Until one day, when the ball is *kicked*. At this moment,everything makes sense to the ball. It understands what it was designed for: it was supposed to be kicked. It looks back at the events that have already taken place and starts connecting the dots. When it was being moved through the air, and when it felt someone applying pressure to it, it experienced feelings of excitement that related to its purpose. The ball now knows what it's been searching for so long….

We gain a degree of satisfaction from applying ourselves toroles that aren't our own profound purpose, but rarely do we have lasting satisfaction. That's not to say that you cannot experience joy – after all, we can always raise our vibration.But we can only feel ultimate fulfillment if we meet the purpose we were made for.

You may find the idea of having a higher purpose to be fantastic,but if you found a smartphone in the middle of a field, you'd assume that someone had dropped it there. You wouldn't think that something so complex was formed naturally by events in nature, over millions of years, without having a designer.

Yet we believe the whole human race, which is far more complex than a smartphone, was produced by a series of mutations and survival of the fittest. Many of us seem to accept that we have no purpose in life, and that we're just another human being in this Universe of billions upon billions of galaxies. However, just like a smartphone, there must surely be a purpose in your existence. When people go through their lives without really believing in a higher purpose, they're not making the most of their existence.

These individuals could go through their whole life just trying to make ends meet. Their purpose in life will always be driven by daily survival, the need to pay the next bill. Of course, bills do matter. We need to pay for food, water, shelter, clothing, and utilities. But do you honestly believe you were put on this planet just to exist in such a manner and then die? Do you truly believe that life is simply about making money?

The Meaning of Life is to Find Your Gift

The Purpose of Your life is to Give is Away

- Pablo Picasso

Just like I used to, many people spend their days working at a job that means nothing to them and living for their two days of freedom each week. During those two days, they'll either do very little or go on a spending spree to make the most of that freedom – as I did by going to a club every weekend. Everyweek they'll look forward to those two days, wishing their precious time away because they want their time away from work – their 'free time' – to come fast. The result is that whole life can go by in a flash. Life is often difficult, and money does give us much more freedom. Nevertheless, have faith that you can serve a purpose for humankind and meet your financial needs. This purpose doesn't have to be something huge – you don't have to be the next Buddha or even the next Ambani.

You must seek to add value, and the only way to do this is by doing something you enjoy with all your heart. This is why passion plays such a big part in living a great life. Not everyone knows what they're passionate about. Spiritual medium Darryl Anka claims to channel a being known asBashar, who advises that following your 'excitement' is the shortest path to realizing what you want; your next step should always be the one you find most exciting. You don't need to justify it, says Bashar, you just need to do it. So take action on whatever it is that truly excites you. Make sure you don't choose something that you label as exciting because you can't think of anything else, or because you think other people will see it as exciting.

Things That Excite You, Aren't RANDOM

They are Connected TO Your Purpose

Follow Them to find your PURPOSE!

So, don't over complicate it by thinking that you need to have it all figured out. And don't be dishonest with yourself and force action on something you feel is unfeasible. For example, if you really like drawing; you could start by creating a website or social media account and sharing some of your work with the world. Don't try to sell your drawings for thousands of pounds right away, particularly if this seems like a long shot to you at this stage. It should be something you're willing to do for free, without any expectation, because it's something you're truly passionate about. If it doesn't excite you, it's not right for you. You don't immediately need to quit your current commitments and put your financial obligations at risk.

What this does mean, though, is that you need to stay curious, stay hungry for positive change, and keep taking steps towards the things that stimulate your mind, body, and soul. Don't worry about which step to take next, or how things will unfold for you. Remember, if you show your excitement to theUniverse, it will give you more things to feel excited about.

Amazing opportunities will follow and help you to discover your path in life, as long as you act on the signs.Small steps are fine because they'll lead to bigger things.Eventually you'll work out a way to make your passion your paycheck. This could be an extension of what you're already doing or, if you're in a profession you dislike, it means you'll eventually be able to give it up and commit to your purposeful-time. You were created with intention. You are here to help, love,assist, save, and entertain. You are here to inspire and put a smile on someone's face.

You are here to make a difference.You wouldn't be on this planet, at this time, if you didn't have something to offer.

There is always a purpose behind your existence, and

when you discover what it is, you will not only

change the dynamics of the world, but also

experience abundance in all areas of your life

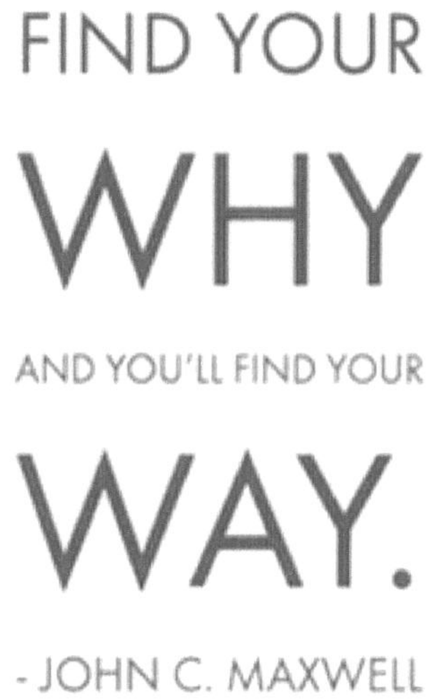

Sh*t no 12

<u>The universal LAW:</u>

The Universe always response to your Vibration

As you think you Vibrate, As you Vibrate You Attract

Beyond the Law of Attraction is the Law of Vibration.

It's the One you learn and apply the ideas around this law, your life will transform. This isn't to say that you'll avoid all difficulties. What you will do OR act though, is find a way to take control and create YOUR life in a similar way.

One of the earliest authors of self-improvement literature is

Napoleon Hill. His 1937 book *Think and Grow Rich* remainsone of the bestselling books of all time, and many of theworld's entrepreneurial gurus praise its guidance to achievingsuccess. Hill's research for his book included interviews with500 successful men and women to find out what they'd doneto attain their success – he then shared the wisdom he'daccumulated from them. Among his conclusions, he claimed:'We are what we are, because of the vibrations of thought which we pick up and register, through the stimuli of our daily environment.' Hill makes many references to the concept of 'vibration' in his book, and you'll see the word 'vibration' today commonly abbreviated to 'vibe'.

Yet many later editions of Hill's book removed any mention of the word 'vibration'. Perhaps the publishers didn't believe the

The world was ready for Hill's concept. Even today, metaphysical

laws related to vibration are under criticism due to a lack of scientific evidence. Despite this, there have been a number of attempts to explain the Law of Vibration. Scientists Dr BruceLipton and author Gregg Braden are among those at the forefront of bridging the gap between science and spirituality.Their ideas on how our thoughts affect our lives support the concept suggested by the Law of Vibration, even if some believe it to be no more than modern pseudoscience.Regardless, for me the Law of Vibration resonates deeply with me, and helps me make sense of life – and I know many others have discovered this, too. I've seen miraculous changes occur from using the Law of Vibration, and whether you become a believer or remain on the other side of the boundary, It Exists…

What you Think, You Become

What you Fell, You Attract

What you Imagine You Create.

Our Life is shaped by our Mind:

WE become what we Think.

-Buddha

<u>*Law of Vibration Means?*</u>

We have heard these lines many times.

"Jo   is

BrahmaandmeinhaiwahihaumaarePindmeinhai"

We have a Whole Universe inside US in small form

To begin with, remember that everything is made up of atoms,and every atom is a little vibration. Therefore, all matter and

Energy is vibrational by nature.If you think of your school, you were taught that solids, liquids and gasses are all different states of matter. The frequency of the vibration at a molecular level defines what state they're in and how they appear to us

In other words, for reality to be perceived, we have to be

vibrationally compatible with it. The human ear, for example,will only hear sound waves that are between 20 and 20,000vibrations per second. This doesn't mean that other soundwaves don't exist; we just can't perceive them. When a dog whistle is blown, the frequency is above the vibrational range of the human ear and therefore doesn't exist to us.

In his book *The Vibrational Universe*,spiritual author

Kenneth James Michael MacLean writes that our five senses,

our thoughts, as well as matter and energy, are *all* vibrational.

He argues that reality is perception defined by vibrational interpretation. Our Universe is clearly a deep sea of vibrational frequencies, meaning that reality is a vibrational ether that's responsive to changes in vibration.If the Universe is responsive to

Change the way you think, feel, speak and act, and you begin to change your world.

To bring an idea into reality, or rather, into your perception,you must match its vibrational frequency. The more 'real' or solid something is to you, the closer you are to it vibrationally.This is why when you truly believe in something and act as if it were already true, you increase the chances of it coming to you in your physical reality. To receive or perceive the reality you wish to have, you must be in energetic harmony with that which you desire. Thismeans that our thoughts, emotions, words, and actions must align with what we really want.

If you want to listen to a specific radio channel you have to tune the receiver to the frequency of that station. This is the only way you can hear it. If you tune in to a different frequency,you'll end up listening to a completely different channel.Once you're in vibrational resonance with something, you begin to attract it into your reality. The best way to identifywhat frequency you're on is through your emotions – your emotions show a true reflection of your energy. Sometimes we can believe we're in a positive state of mind or taking good actions, but deep down we know we're not; we're just pretending. If we pay attention to our emotions, we can see the true nature of our vibration and therefore what we're attracting into our life. If we feel good, we'll think good thoughts, and as a result we'll take positive actions.

<u>THE UNIVERSAL LAWS</u>

The Law of Divine Oneness

EVERYTHING IS CONNECTED

The Law of Vibration

EVERYTHING HAS A UNIQUE VIBRATIONAL FREQUENCY

The Law of Attraction

WHAT IS LIKE UNTO ITSELF IS DRAWN

The Law of Correspondence

AS ABOVE SO BELOW

The Law of Action

MANIFESTATION REQUIRES ALIGNED ACTION

The Law of Perpetual Transmutation of Energy

ENERGY IS ALWAYS MOVING AND CHANGING

The Law of Compensation

EVERY RIGHT ACTION HAS A REWARD

The Law of Relativity

IT'S ALL RELATIVE

The Law of Polarity

THERE ARE TWO SIDES TO EVERYTHING

The Law of Cause and Effect

EVERY ACTION HAS A CONSEQUENCE

The Law of Rhythm

NOTHING IS PERMANENT

The Law of Gender

MANIFESTATION REQUIRES A BALANCE OF BOTH ENERGIES

Sh*t no 13

<u>EGO vs SOUL</u>:

Our soul and our ego are both part of who we are, and we can look at them as opposite aspects of ourselves that coexist and come to the forefront when we need them, depending on the situation that we're in. When we think of ego vs soul it's easy to see one as good (the soul) and one as bad (the ego) but that isn't *really* the case.

Ego is just as necessary as the soul is when we need it, and it's what sets us apart as humans because as far as we know, no other animal has an ego in the way that we do.

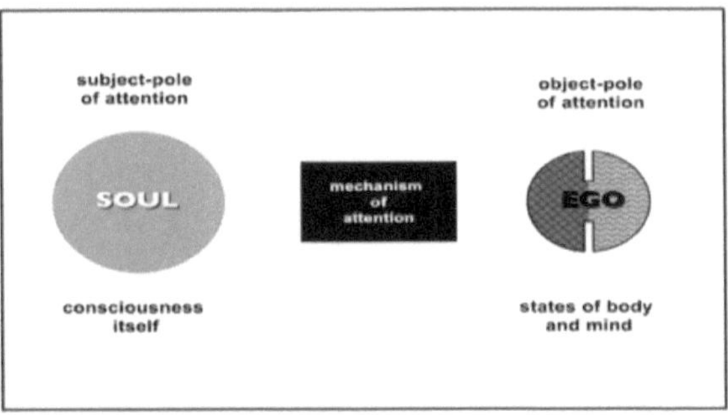

Human Operating System

Just as a computer and a phone have an operating system, so does our own awareness. The twin poles of attention represent the basic operating system of human awareness

Twin Poles of Attention

The twin poles of attention are the subject-pole and the object-pole At the object-pole is everything we are aware of, including thoughts, emotions, beliefs, perceptions, memories, hopes, ideas, self-image, etc. At the subject-pole of attention is consciousness itself.

Opposite Polarity

The ego and the soul are located at opposite poles of attention. The ego is identified with the object-pole of attention (states of body and mind), and the soul is identified with the subject-pole of attention (consciousness itself).

The ego and soul are located at opposite poles of attention.

Ego

The ego is your body-mind self, or your false self. The ego is founded on identification with your body and mind at the object-pole of attention. The ego exercises IQ and EQ but has no access to SQ.

Soul

The soul is your existential self, or your true self. The soul is founded on identification with consciousness itself at the subject-pole of attention. The soul exercises IQ and EQ with SQ.

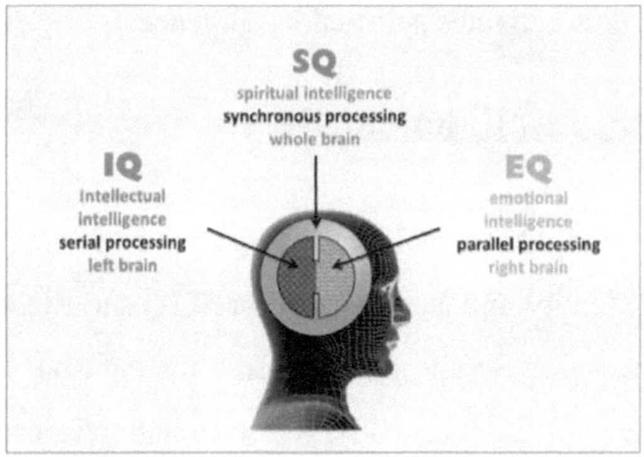

Different Purposes

The ego and the soul use IQ and EQ for different purposes. The ego uses IQ and EQ for personal gain, in the constant search for compensation for the inevitable dissatisfaction of being the ego.

But the intelligence of the soul has a different purpose. SQ uses IQ and EQ for the benefit of all, to express the native qualities of consciousness itself, which are experienced at the subject-pole of attention in moments of presence, in the form of wisdom, compassion, integrity, joy, love, creativity, and peace.

Spiritual intelligence shifts from ego to soul at the opposite pole of attention.

From Ego to Soul

The essence of spiritual intelligence is the shift from false self to true self, from ego to soul, at the opposite pole of attention. The SQ portal is a simple three-step process that rapidly shifts from ego to soul, and thus activates spiritual intelligence.

Spiritual Intelligence

Spiritual intelligence replaces the ego with the soul as the seat of personal identity and as the governor of IQ and EQ. Thus, spiritual intelligence uses IQ and EQ, not from the ego, but from your true self as the soul. Consequently, SQ lives with wisdom, compassion, and integrity, which is the ultimate form of fulfillment.

I will try to explain in simpler terms,

What is ego?

"Ego" is the Latin word for "I", and I think this definition can give you a pretty good idea of what the ego means on its own. The ego is who we are in our minds - it's composed of conscious thoughts and beliefs, labels, and our sense of identity. The ego is helpful when it comes to making some decisions because it's good at weighing up consequences and outcomes and seeing things objectively. It is also a motivating force that can help us thrive in today's society - it often gets the job done, for whatever reason that may be. It is also what determines our own perspective of the external world, though this can often be flawed because it is so easily affected by our own emotions and past experiences, rather than the true reality. And unlike the soul, it is mostly self-serving, thinking of your own wants and needs, as opposed to the collective. But as I said before, I think the ego gets a bad rep, and

there are times when this self-serving force is necessary and dare I say it, a *good* thing.Interestingly, some yogic cultures define the ego in three parts (much like Freud's definitions of the ego, superego and id).

According to Art of Living, these are the 3 aspects of our ego:

- **The Tamasic ego**: self-destructive, blind
- **The Rejasic ego**: self-centered
- **The Sattvic ego**: creative and protective

So, if this is true, our aim should **not** be to get rid of the ego entirely, but to **move towards the Sattvic ego** over the other types, and to use it to our advantage when it serves us for good.

What is the soul?

In contrast, the soul is pretty much the polar opposite of everything the ego represents. The soul self doesn't rely on logical decision making, but instead allows itself to be **guided by** intuition or signs from the Universe.

This is the part of us that exists when the ego self has taken a step back, which is often described as a **"flow state"** where external constructs like time no longer exist. The soul might be regarded as your **"true nature"**, since this is the essence of who you are, without the influence of labels, expectations or judgments - it just *is*.

Soul over Ego

When they're in balance, the soul and the ego are able to perfectly coexist- it's only when one takes dominance over the other in a situation that it is not suited to that becomes problematic. And contrary to what some spiritual teachers will tell you, **the aim isn't to squash the ego completely**, because the soul self can equally take over and be unhelpful in some situations. Think about being in a life or death situation - the ego is the force that is going to help you with problem solving to get out of that situation safely, ultimately leading to your survival. In the same situation the soul would be pretty useless at this level of problem solving, and it wouldn't come with the same sense of urgency to save your life. It would however be useful in keeping you calm and preventing your emotions from taking over completely, which would otherwise likely result in you being paralyzed by fear and being able to take no action at all.

The aim is therefore to find balance between the two, and to recognize when one has taken over when it's unnecessary and potentially problematic. Admittedly, due to the way our societies have become, with a focus on material possessions and instant feedback loops in the form of social media apps, it is much more likely for the ego to take center stage in unwanted situations than vice versa.

So how do we learn to take a step back and choose soul over ego in these situations?

Spotting when the ego is in charge is the most important step in choosing your soul over it. If you don't know when the ego has taken hold, how can you know to let go of it? It can be really difficult to spot when our ego has come to the forefront, since it is a powerful driving force in all of us, and many of us live our lives entirely through our Egos without ever questioning it.

But once we learn to spot the ego in charge, we can intentionally choose to push it to the side and choose our soul instead, when we don't think that the ego is serving us. And the good news is that it only takes once for you to say no to your ego, and then it will get easier and easier

How to spot when your ego is in charge ?

(and isn't serving you)

You often **feel consumed by your emotions**, particularly ones of anger, hurt or disappointmentYou have a **more extrinsic sense of worth**, meaning that you get your validation from outside sources like material possessions or other people's opinions of you

You **"overthink" things,** and **struggle to make decisions** due to heavily analyzing the potential outcomes.You are **highly critical** of yourself and others, and make objective judgements

You **see things in black and white**, gravitate towards labels and feel the need to compartmentalize things into boxes. You're **easily hurt/angered/disappointed** when things don't go your way or you don't get the outcome you expectedYou **take other people's actions and projections personally**, even when they're not.

How to spot when your soul is in charge

(and is serving you)

You **don't take other people's actions or decisions to heart**, knowing that they are not a reflection of you and are projections of their own internal stateYou are more readily **able to practice forgiveness** and **let go of the past**, preferring not to dwell on things that are no longer in your controlYou have a desire to better yourself, but your **self-worth does not depend on achieving goals Our sense of self-worth is constant** and isn't affected by the opinions of others or the acquisition of material possessions

You feel **less attached to outcomes** and are **able to "go with the flow" or "trust your gut"**You **don't feel a need to fit into a particular box or label**, and instead listen to what you are called to, even when that changesYou **lose yourself** and a sense of time when doing things you enjoy. You **feel called to go after your own interests and desires,** even when they go against the grain of what is "normal" or "expected of you"**Life feels more effortless**, like the Universe is gently guiding you forward

Ego vs soul relationships: what they look like

Ego Focused Relationship	Soul Focused Relationship
Getting into frequent arguments because of differing points of view	Celebrating each other's differences, using as opportunities to learn & grow together
Comparing your relationships to	Knowing your relationship is

others (whether online or in real life)	unique and embracing its positive aspects
Letting other opinions govern your relationships	Knowing what is right for you
Feeling pressured to achieve relationship milestones by certain times or age benchmarks	Doing things at your own pace and trusting the journey
Getting into relationships in order to feel emotionally validated and worthy	Learning to love yourself and allowing anything else to be an addition
Wanting to fix or change others	Knowing what is and isn't aligned with you
Not wanting to leave a relationship because of previous expectations or fears of wasted time	Knowing when it's right to leave a relationship that is no longer serving you
Getting into a relationship that isn't suited due to low self esteem	Knowing your worth and declining relationships with those who aren't suited
Being a people pleaser and doing things to gain approval	Being able to say no when things don't feel right
Having relationships for selfish reasons and hurting others	Having valuable relationships with connection as the

primary focus

Ego vs Soul quotes

These are some powerful ego vs soul quotes that can help you further understand the difference between ego, and the soul.

"Ego finds what it wants in words, the soul finds what it needs in silence."   *- Unknown*

"When the ego dies, the soul awakes." - Mahatma Gandhi

The finish line is for the ego, the journey is for the soul."

Ego v/s Soul relationships:

In my opinion, relationships are one of the most affected areas of our life and the most likely to suffer from an imbalance of soul and ego. Having experienced many ego-based relationships, I know how detrimental they can be for your own growth and wellbeing. Recognising when the ego has taken over in your relationships in unhealthy ways, whether from yourself or the other party (or both),

is essential in shifting towards a more healthy relationship or making the decision to walk away.

Ego says once everything falls into place, I will find

peace.

Soul says once I find peace,

Everything will fall into place."

When it comes to ego vs soul, the soul is often the desired state in many situations. But **don't take this as the ego being the enemy -** there are many situations in which the ego is a beneficial state to be in - it's about recognizing when it's unneeded and when to push it aside in favor of the soul. **Switch your focus towards shifting towards a more Sattvic ego**, and calling in your soul self when you feel you may be getting too ego dominant. It's a process, so don't beat yourself up when you slip into your ego self often

Date your Ego --- Marry Your Soul

Enjoy the journey and understand

that it's all about finding balance.

Sh*t no 14

<u>Love your Uniqueness:</u>

I Love these unique words

"APRICITY"

Which means the Warmth of the Sun in Winters

"AVIOTHIC"

The Strong Desire to be up in the air To FLY

"MOROSIS"

The stupidest of Stupidness

Just be like Apricity in someone's life and

Aviothic in desire be the Uniqueness in You

And Morosis to be as stupid and childish

To chase your dreams and happiness.

As young kids, we're regularly listening that we're all individuals and should have no shame in being ourselves. We're encouraged to pursue our wildest dreams! After some time as we grow, our world of possibility shrinks. People say, 'Yes, be yourself... but not like we thought in our childhood days!' The deep meaning of "You can be anything in the world" ... is actually to take the right path as per society ideology. In psychology, the concept of 'social proof' suggests that people like to follow the crowd. If everyone else is doing it, you assume it's the right thing to do. Other people influence your actions more than you realize. For example, if you had to pick between Science, Arts and Commerce, most of the colleges filled up Science stream first then commerce, if no option left then parents ask their children to take Arts, it is their perception that Arts is for no use, But the Truth is totally opposite of it. Society's thinking has been like this for years this way and we can't alone change it. I scored good marks in SSC, and I loved Psychology and Geography more so I chose ARTS. But just because everyone else is doing it does *not* mean it's right.

Slavery used to be legal, but now nearly everyone would agree that it's inhumane, degrading, and immoral. Start to question your actions. Why do you do what you do, and choose what you choose? Are you doing what you really think is right, or are you following the crowd?

Fear and scarcity are commonly used to control society. I've Known many people who, instead of living the life they have chosen, have lived the life they were told to by others in the form of well-meaning guidance and support. And while some people *want* what's best for you, they may not *understand what's* best for you. They may also make decisions for you based on fear that's been passed on to them by someone else.If you discover your choices are frequently dictated by the views of others,you know you're relinquishing control over your life. Without control, we panic and end up in low vibrational states, such as anxiety. Ultimately, we end up having no control over how much joy we experience, as we become slaves to other people's opinions.

But you shouldn't feel like you're living someone else's beliefs. You shouldn't feel like you have to meet everyone else's expectations or live your life a certain way to gain their approval. You shouldn't feel like you have to shy away from being who you really are, from your uniqueness. Life Shouldn't feel limiting.

Someone once said ye that, "*Kutte Bhoke Ga, par hathi chalta rahega*"The truth is, either way, you're going to be judged by the people, whether you live life on your own terms or on others they will say or comment.

So find your Uniqueness and lead your life as you want.

Authenticity is rare these days, & many of our actions are the suggestion or replication of someone else. Without drawing you into paranoia, we're easily reprogrammed to satisfy the needs of others. Don't let your individuality get taken away from you, just so you can fit in with the rest of society. *Embrace your uniqueness.* Are you considered weird? Awesome! This is only because most people are living inside an imaginary box and you don't fit in it; and we're led to believe that when you don't fit society's needs, something is wrong with you. Who wants to be bound by a box that isn't even there? Not me! Freedom has no constraints. We can always improve ourselves and grow as individuals. We can step out of our comfort zone and challenge ourselves. But society often makes us feel like we're wrong for just being ourselves.

Its my personal experience of leaving a highly prestigious job in one of the top 5 MNCs in India. Despite being in a manager position and holding a high designation, felt compelled to leave the job and pursue something that aligned with their inner desires and values. Others did not understand the author's decision wholeheartedly but supported my family in spite of the job which was highly respected and prestigious.

I had a mixed feeling. I was confused, frightened but happy and peace, it was not an easy decision to make. However, I chose to follow my own path, even if it went against societal expectations and norms. I have faced criticism, judgment from others for making this decision.

Overall, I'm highlighting the importance of making decisions that align with personal values and desires, even if they go against societal expectations or norms. It also suggests that following one's own path may require courage and may involve facing criticism or judgment from others. However, the potential rewards of pursuing personal fulfillment and happiness are worth the risks and challenges that may come with it.

My current emotional state of being happy and content with the decision I made to leave job and pursue a path that aligned with my personal desires and values. I likely feels a sense of fulfillment and satisfaction from having taken control of my life and worked hard to make their decision a success. Choice is and will always be yours my dear friend, You absolutely cannot blame anyone else for it.

They will call you quiet because you're

perfectly happy in silence.

They will call you weak because you

avoid conflict and drama.

They will call you obsessed for being

passionate about the things you love.

They will call you rude for not

engaging in social pleasantries.

They will call you arrogant for having self-respect.

They will call you boring for not being extroverted.

They will call you wrong for having different beliefs.

They will call you shy when you choose

not to interact in small talk.

They will call you weird because you choose

not to conform to societal trends.

They will call you fake for trying

your best to remain positive.

They will call you a loner because you're

comfortable being on your own.

They will call you lost for not following

the same route as others.

They will call you a geek for being

a knowledge-seeker.

They will call you ugly for not

looking like celebrities.

They will call you dumb for not being an academic.

They will call you crazy for thinking

differently from others.

They will call you cheap for

knowing value for money.

They will call you disloyal for distancing

yourself from negative people.

- Good vibes Good Life (Vex King)

Stop listing the outside noise, deep dive into yourself for the Answers you are searching for… Because only you know your A-Z story inside out…

Choose your Uniqueness because you have <u>KEFI</u> inside you.

KE-FI is a concept from Greek culture that refers to the feeling of joy and contentment that arises from simple and meaningful experiences. It is often associated with feelings of well-being, satisfaction, and happiness.

The concept of KE-FI can be applied to various aspects of life, such as enjoying a good meal with friends, participating in a community activity, or taking a leisurely walk in nature.KE-FI is believed to stem from a sense of connectedness to others and to the world around us, as well as a feeling of being present in the moment and fully engaged in the experience.

In Greek culture, KE-FI is often associated with music,dance, and celebration, as these activities are believed to foster a sense of connection and joy among individuals. The concept of KE-FI has also been adopted and celebrated in other cultures around the world, as people recognize the value of simple and meaningful experiences in promoting happiness and well-being.

KE-FI is a concept that emphasizes the importance of finding joy and contentment in everyday experiences, and of cultivating a sense of connectedness to others and to the world around us.

Are you? Ask Yourself ...

Sh*t no 15

That 1%:

The "1% Rule" is if you can just consistently and persistently be 1% better at what you do each day, over the course of a year or a decade you will make significant progress. Specifically:

Why and how it works.

When you study why some people achieve a lot with their careers, you'll find those on the top of the mountain make ongoing, steady progress in doing meaningful work all the time. They harness consistency and time to produce maximum results. The key is to make daily micro-progress towards your goals, rather than expecting major breakthroughs to materialize.

The 1% Rule — Applying the 1% Code.

To apply the 1% Rule long enough to move the needle in your own life and career, you need a code — a foundational philosophy of virtues and values. This will ground you and guide you and motivate you to endure even when stress and chaos arise.

So how do you motivate &organize yourself to be 1% better every day? It comes down to 6 principles which make up The 1% Code:

You would logically be the amount to a 365% lift in results over the course of a year, but author Tommy Baker points outcompounding will boost those results even more. I added one more step that is Marketing. If you consistently do one percent better over the course of a year, you can potentially boost what you do 30-times or more.

1. <u>Fall In Love With The Process:</u>

It's about falling in love with the process. Once we do, we're able to put our limited physical, mental, and emotional energy into it with everything we've got. The process is the metamorphosis of who you've been to who you're becoming.Without this foundational principle, we'll crumble. Inherently, the process involves challenging moments, breakthroughs, and everything in between. If we expect these to happen, they won't divert us, and we'll keep sharpening our sword every single day.

2. <u>Do It Every Single Day</u>

As long as we're moving 1% daily, we harness the incredible powers of the rule. It's less about the size and duration of the progress but more about the fact that we're making progress that counts.

There are things you and I already do every single day because they're important. We shower, we brush our teeth, we tell our significant others we love them, we fire up our computer, etc. At first glance, committing to do something every single day can seem daunting, but it's the opposite. It takes the pressure off and allows us to flex the muscle of consistency.

3: Celebrate Your Commitment

A crucial part of the code is celebrating our wins, even the small, seemingly insignificant ones. Emphasis is on the word seemingly,because the size & scope of the win doesn't matter—it's the fact you won, & it must be acknowledged. Every single day, we celebrate a win we experience as we use the 1% Rule. These micro-wins create the momentum & clarity required to get us to the more expansive wins and outcomes we're chasing. They force us to open our awareness, &we feed our inner hero instead of our inner critic. They remind us to not judge ourselves &instead appreciate our growth.

4: Track Your Metrics & Data

Although this part of the code won't light you up with inspiration, it's essential to clearly see the inputs and outputs of our work. Without tracking, we live in a fantasy, which makes decision-makinga nightmare.If we don't have accurate data, our emotions and feelings start to take over, and we base our decisions off those.

While emotions & feelings serve a purpose, they're always changing by default and can't be relied on. Our feelings &emotions are like the ocean tide, while data and metrics are more like mountains. Peter Drucker famously said: "If you can't measure it, you can't improve it." In this context, it's never been more relevant and true.

5: Master Your Craft

Regardless of what your craft may be, the mindset and components of mastery are proven to transcend skill and scope. While the 1% Rule will be used for every part of your life, your ability to focus on a specific craft will separate you from your competition.

Deliberate practice. It's easy to practice a skill & do what we're good at. Can you instead spend the time on what challenges you?

Invest thousands of hours. Mastery takes time, there's no way around it. Expect to invest in thousands of hours to deliberate practice as you sharpen your skills.

Long-term consistency. It's easy to invest time and effort in a skill when it's new. Once you start to become decent at it, it can become boring. Embracing this and pushing past to a place where you endure will make you invaluable to any marketplace.

6: Marketing is the heart of success:

Marketing doesn't always relate to products or services which we sell or purchase.Showcasing our self is also a form of marketing, if someone is working in a firm as an employee also does marketing but they feel it's just they are letting them to know who you are and what you know in your Resume, but actually You tend to learn workplace skills (sometimes known as soft skills) through experience, and you can apply them to a number of different tasks and roles. In marketing, there are six workplace skills that will be important to develop and sharpen throughout your career.

1. Creativity

Marketing involves working with ideas—and improving them in order to reach new and existing customers—so all marketing roles require creativity to some extent. While some roles, like copywriter or social media coordinator, may demand more creativity on a daily basis than others, having a strong creative sensibility will serve you well in your marketing career.

What this looks like:

- Producing short, innovative videos for a new social media campaign

- Identifying a new way to conduct market research so your team learns something new about competitors

- Making PPTS, MIS report in your own way to describe reports better and simpler

- Finding a new program or tool that will better track customer engagement

2. Research

Marketers develop savvy campaigns that encourage customers to *do* something or buy a product or add new services to their account. Knowing how to conduct both qualitative and quantitative research can help you find data that may help inform your team's specific efforts.

What this looks like:

- Using social media listening tools, to understand what customers are saying directly or indirectly about a product to improve more

- Conducting market research on a major competitor's products

- Doing keyword research to make sure your content aligns with user intent

3. Listening

In addition to the research that you conduct about customers, it's equally important to listen to the feedback they offer. What pain points do your customers experience? What do they most enjoy about your latest products? Listening requires a good degree of empathy and can train you to be more flexible by staying open to suggestions that shift the course of your marketing efforts.

What this looks like:

- Paying attention to the comments customers post on social media

- Tracking site metrics to see how much time users are spending on various pages

- Reviewing surveys and other qualitative data for insights

4. Communication

Marketers must be excellent communicators in a few different ways: with audiences, with team members, and with major stakeholders and company leaders. Being able to clearly and efficiently communicate with these different groups can not only help you succeed in your various tasks but may also help you avoid any problems that arise from poor communication.

What this looks like:

- Responding to customers' complaints with respect and empathy

- Drafting emails to marketing team members about an

upcoming campaign launch

- Leading a presentation to company stakeholders about annual results

And here comes success in your life in various form. The hard part, in my opinion, is to keep reminding yourself what you're trying to do. It's also a bit tricky sometimes to definitively say you've done one percent better than yesterday, especially if you're dealing with issues which have no hard and fast metrics or measures. But the basic concept that you try and move forward every day rather than falling for the myths is powerful and practical. That 1 % improvement required daily involvement (Time) that is called Consistency and making habits and designing your path.

Sh*t no 16

Habit and consistency

Habit and consistency are two different but related concepts. Habits are the most important and crucial part of life to be successful, I have exclusively designed the course where I make people form the habits with my 9-step powerful formula and how to overcome your comfort zone to achieve consistency, tried and tested proven life changing Formula .

A habit is a behavior that is repeated regularly and often automatically in response to specific triggers or cues. Habits are formed through consistent repetition and reinforcement, where the brain learns to associate a specific behavior with a particular context or stimulus. The idea is that by repeating a behavior over time, it becomes ingrained in our daily routine and requires less conscious effort to perform.

Consistency, on the other hand, refers to the quality of being dependable, reliable, & predictable in one's actions. Being consistent means following through on commitments, showing up at the same time every day, and sticking to a routine or schedule. Consistency is about maintaining a steady pattern of behavior over time, rather than sporadically doing something.In essence, habits and consistency are related because consistent repetition is necessary to form a habit. But while habits are about automating a specific behavior, consistency is more about maintaining a stable pattern of behavior over time, regardless of whether that behavior is a habit or not.

Habits - Bit By Bit makes habits. This is a key part of our daily lives, and research suggests that as much as 40-45% of our daily actions are habitual. Habits can be formed through a process called "habituation," where the brain learns to associate a specific behavior with a particular context or stimulus. Over time, this association becomes automatic and requires less conscious effort to perform the behavior. Habits are behaviors that we repeatedly perform in response to certain cues or triggers, often without conscious awareness or deliberate intention. Habits can be both beneficial and detrimental to our lives, depending on their nature.

Habits can be positive or negative, depending on the behavior and its impact on our lives. Positive habits like regular exercise, healthy eating, and consistent sleep patterns can have significant benefits for our physical and mental health. Negative habits like smoking, excessive drinking, and procrastination can have harmful effects on our health, relationships, and overall well-being.

While habits can be challenging to break, research suggests that it is possible to establish new habits or replace existing ones with more positive behaviors. This often involves consciously identifying the behavior you want to change, establishing a specific goal or plan, and tracking your progress over time. By doing so, you can reinforcePositive behaviors & gradually replace negative habits with more positive ones.

I'm sharing a few powerful formulas to build Habit from my course:

Pretty much everyone on the planet wants to build better habits — both personal and professional. Few of them may want to leave a bad habit as well, However, change is hard. There's a painful gap between expectations and reality most of the time. That's where Tiny Habits comes in.

"Tiny Habits" is a habit formation methodology which aligns with how human psychology actually works. The essence of the Tiny Habits approach to behavior design is:

Forming a habit requires effort and consistency, but it is a powerful way to create positive changes in your life. Here are some steps to help you form a habit:

1. <u>Start small</u>: Choose a habit that is simple and easy to do. Starting with a small habit can help you build momentum and increase your chances of success.

2. <u>Set a goal</u>: Decide on a specific goal and a timeframe for achieving it. This will help you stay focused and motivated.

3. <u>Create a routine</u>: Choose a specific time and place to do your habit. This will help you create a routine and make it

easier to remember to do your habit.

4. <u>Track your progress:</u> Keep track of your progress and celebrate your successes. This will help you stay motivated and build momentum.

5. <u>Stay committed</u>: Stick with your habit even when it gets difficult. It takes time to form a habit, but with consistency and commitment, it will become easier over time.

6. <u>Reward yourself:</u> Celebrate your successes along the way. This will help you stay motivated and reinforce the habit you are trying to form.

Remember that forming a habit takes time and effort, so be patient and keep at it. Over time, your habit will become automatic, and you will enjoy the benefits of your efforts.

Consistency :Also a key factor in achieving success in many

areas of life, including personal relationships, work, and hobbies. Here are some ways in which consistency can contribute to success:

Overall, consistency can be a powerful tool in achieving success, but it requires sustained effort and dedication over time. By staying focused on your goals and maintaining consistent action, you can build momentum and achieve the success you desire.

Consistency is an important trait when it comes to achieving your goals and making progress in your life. Here are some tips to help you be more consistent:

1. Set realistic goals: Choose goals that are achievable and realistic. This will help you avoid setting yourself up for failure and discouragement.

2. Make a plan: Create a plan for how you will achieve your goals. Break down your goals into smaller steps and create a timeline for achieving each step.

3. Schedule time: Schedule time for working on your goals. This could be a specific time of day or a certain number of hours per week.

4. Prioritize: Make your goals a priority. Avoid distractions and focus on what is most important to you.

5. Stay motivated: Keep your motivation high by reminding yourself of why you want to achieve your goals. Celebrate your successes along the way, and don't be too hard on yourself if you experience setbacks.

6. Be accountable: Tell someone else about your goals and ask them to hold you accountable. This can help you stay on track and motivated.

7. Practice discipline: Consistency requires discipline. Make a habit of doing what you need to do, even when you don't feel like it.

<u>Habits are the compound interest of self-improvement</u>.

Remember that consistency is a habit, and like any habit, it takes time and effort to develop. Start small and build up your consistency over time. With practice, you will find it easier to stay consistent and achieve your goals.

Sh*t no 17

<u>Going Deep: GRIT</u>

Passion And Perseverance

Skills are Inexpensive… Passion is Priceless

"Whatever makes you feel The Sun from the inside out chase that"

-Gemma Troy

Love What You Do OR Do What You Love

Life Is Greater If You Live With Purpose.

When You Find A Meaningful Reason For

Doing What You Do, You Will Feel Complete.

Passion and perseverance are two important qualities that can help you achieve your goals and lead a fulfilling life.

Passion is the intense, driving force that motivates you to pursue your goals and dreams. It's the feeling of excitement and enthusiasm that comes from doing something that you love and are deeply committed to. Passion can help you overcome obstacles and setbacks, because it gives you the drive to keep going even when things get tough.

Perseverance, on the other hand, is the quality of persistence and determination in the face of challenges and setbacks. It's the ability to keep working towards your goals even when progress is slow or difficult. Perseverance is what enables you to keep going even when you feel like giving up, and to push through obstacles and challenges in order to achieve your objectives.Together, passion and perseverance can be a powerful combination that can help you achieve great things in life. By pursuing yourpassions with determination& persistence, you can overcome challenges and setbacks and achieve the success & fulfillment that you desire.

Here's and example : Yug is a trust-fund-baby whose dad has set him up for life. He was born with an IQ of 140, attended the best schools, but still has trouble committing to projects. Sia was born into modest circumstances. She's intelligent enough without being the next Einstein but has a work ethic that allows her to knuckle down and fight through any obstacles that stand in her way.

Who would you rather be: Yug or Sia?

Are you better off being a simpleminded person who works hard, or a talented person who takes it easy? Angela Duckworth has studied hard to find the answers to this question, in search of the qualities that make for an extraordinary life. And she's found a compelling answer: the key to success is what she calls "Grit". It is a mixture of both Passion & Perseverance to get the job done.

We just learnt the magic number for success seems to be 10,000 hrs of commitment to a path. But that's obviously a long time. You might get bored, you might get distracted by the shiny new object that crosses your vision, or it might get too hard, and you throw in the towel. Grit is what can keep you on track.

It turns out the hard workers beat the naturally gifted across a wide variety of domains:

"Without effort, your talent is nothing more than unmet potential. Without effort, your skill is nothing more than what you could have done but you didn't."

Passion and Perseverance for long term Goal is called GRIT

-Inspired by: **Grit**, *by Angela Duckworth*

In Psychology GRIT is a positive character trait based on an individual's passion for a particular long-term goal or end state coupled with powerful motivation to achieve this object.

<u>These are several Key aspect of GRIT to explain further</u>:

1. Perseverance: Grit involves a high level of perseverance, which means that individuals with grit are able to maintain their effort and focus on their goals despite obstacles, setbacks, & failures.

2. Passion: Gritty individuals have a strong sense of passion for their goals, which provides them with the motivation and drive to work towards them over a long period of time.

3. Resilience: Individuals with grit are able to bounce back from failures and setbacks, and are able to learn from these experiences in order to improve and continue making progress.

4. Self-discipline: Gritty individuals have a strong sense of self-discipline, which allows them to stay focused on their goals and resist the temptation to give up or become distracted.

5. Growth mindset: Gritty individuals have a growth mindset, meaning that they view challenges and failures as

opportunities for growth and improvement, rather than as indications of their inherent abilities.

6. Long-term focus: Individuals with grit have a long-term focus, and are able to delay gratification in order to achieve their goals over time.

Overall, these aspects of grit are closely interconnected, and work together to enable individuals to persist in the face of challenges and achieve their long-term goals.

PASSION – Excellence versus Perfection

(Perfection is excellence's somewhat pernicious cousin)

(Excellent is an Attitude, not an Endgame)

Try to be Excellent in what you do, rather not wait for perfection for long to start your action.

Despite the perseverance and passion measures being the clear leading indicators of success, the world is still obsessed with talent. We think of 'talent' as being some innate special ability we're born with. But talent isn't an indication of your skill level,

it's merely the rate at which you can develop skills. Talent

doesn't mean we're already good at something – it just means we can get better at something quicker.

Talent x Effort = Skill

Skill x Effort = Achievement

In these equations, effort counts twice. Applying effort to your talents gives you skills, then more effort is required to turn those skills into achievements. Without applied effort, that natural talent is meaningless.

previously though I was a pretty hard-working creature and assumed that I would score reasonably high and pursued a good number of side hustles, and I kept on working and learning and releasing videos

Sh*t no 18

<u>Shifting Focous</u>

The idea is that "always be appreciative" what you have increase what you want" can be interpreted in a few different ways, but one possible explanation is that by cultivating gratitude for what we already have, we develop a mindset of abundance and positive energy that attracts more good things into our lives.

When we focus on what we lack or what we want, we can create a sense of scarcity or lack in our minds, which can lead to negative emotions such as frustration, anxiety, or envy. However, by shifting our focus to what we already have and expressing gratitude for it, we can create a sense of abundance and positivity that attracts more good things into our lives.

In this sense, the act of appreciating what we have can help us to clarify our desires and intentions, and to open ourselves up to the possibilities of growth and abundance. It can also help us to cultivate a positive mindset and a sense of joy and fulfillment in the present moment, rather than constantly chasing after more or better things.

Being grateful or showing appreciation for something or someone. It is the ability to recognize and value the good qualities, actions, or gifts of others, and to express gratitude or thanks in response.

Appreciation is an important quality in building and maintaining positive relationships with others, as it shows that we value and acknowledge their contributions or efforts. It can also lead to greater satisfaction and happiness in our own lives, as we focus on the positive aspects of our experiences and relationships rather than dwelling on the negative.

Here are some more ways to express gratitude:

1. Write a thank-you note: Take the time to write a

handwritten note expressing your gratitude for something someone has done for you. This can be a thoughtful and personal way to show your appreciation.

2. Verbalize your gratitude: Tell the person directly how much you appreciate what they've done for you. You can express your gratitude in person, over the phone, or in a video call.

3. Practice gratitude journaling: Write.

Feeling Grateful

Feeling grateful is an emotion that arises when we recognize and appreciate the good things in our lives. It is a positive and uplifting feeling that can help to improve our mood, increase our sense of well-being, and foster a greater sense of connection and empathy with others.

"Shifting your focus from bad things happening in your life" can be a challenge, but there are some steps you can take to help improve the situation. Here are some suggestions:

1. Take a break: Sometimes, stepping away from a situation can help you gain perspective and clarity. Take a break and do something that makes you feel good, such as going for a walk, listening to music, or

spending time with friends or family.

2. Practice self-care: Taking care of yourself is important when dealing with a difficult situation. This includes getting enough sleep, eating well, and engaging in activities that make you feel good.

3. Identify what you can control: There may be aspects of the situation that you can't control, but there are likely some things that you can control. Identify what those things are and focus your energy on them.

4. Set small goals: Setting small goals can help you feel a sense of accomplishment and progress, even when dealing with a challenging situation. Break down larger tasks into smaller, more manageable steps.

5. Seek support: Talk to someone you trust about what you're going through. This can be a friend, family member, or professional. Having support can help you feel less alone and can provide you with new perspectives on the situation.

6. Practice gratitude: Despite the difficulties you're facing, try to find things in your life that you're grateful for. Focusing on the positive can help shift your perspective and improve your mood.

Remember that dealing with difficult situations takes time and effort. Be patient with yourself and try to focus on small steps that you can take to improve the situation.

Truly speaking, Our MOOD is the Biggest Culprit for all the mess in our life, humeachanahilagta to hum bahut kuchaisakartehai jo ki sahinaihota fir bhi hum kartehai,

For example – Sad hai to aur sad song dhoonddhoondk suntehai, iss pain aur badhtahai, kamnaihota.

Gussahai to aur Gussabharibaatekartehai aur pin point kartehai, aur chillachilla k boltehaijissa aur heart beat badtahai

Kisis k baato ko buralaga to bar baarwahitape recorder cassetteapnedimag me play karterehtahai, "Usnemujheaisa bola kaisa, kyamaisach me aisihoon aur apnaaap pe aap khud doubt kartehai aur gussa ho jatehai, aur apka mood kharab ho jatahai aur bhi. Sachkahiyakartehaina hum sab aisa…

Aur bhi bahut sare example mil jayegaapke life me kyo ki hum karte to wahihai sab ek hi pattern par chalterehtahai.

Our mood can be influenced by many factors, including our environment, physical state, and our thoughts. Here are some strategies you can use to help change your mood:Here are some of mine

1. Exercise: Exercise releases endorphins, which are natural mood-boosters. Engaging in physical activity, even for a short period of time, can help improve your mood.

2. Listen to music: Music can have a powerful effect on our mood. Listening to uplifting music can help improve your mood and decrease feelings of sadness

or anxiety.

3. Practice gratitude: Focusing on the things you are grateful for can help shift your perspective and improve your mood. Take some time to write down or think about the things that you appreciate in your life.

4. Connect with others: Spending time with friends or family, or even just talking to someone on the phone, can help improve your mood and decrease feelings of loneliness.

5. Practice mindfulness: Mindfulness involves paying attention to the present moment without judgment. Engaging in mindfulness practices, such as meditation or deep breathing, can help you feel more calm and centered.

6. Engage in a hobby: Doing something that you enjoy, such as reading, painting, or playing a musical instrument, can help improve your mood and decrease stress.

7. Seek professional help: If you're struggling with your mood and finding it difficult to improve, it's important to seek professional help. A therapist or counselor can provide you with the tools and support you need to improve your mood and overall mental health.

Most of the cases which I m handling and coming through is the feeling of loneliness, depression, akelaapan, emotionally empty, koi naihaijiskoapnadardbaat sake, koi naihaisamajnewalamujhe, there is no end to my pain, khoklaapanlagtahai, sab kuchhai fir bhikuchnaihai, bus sab karrahehai par khali pan haietc…. aur kabikabi ye sab pain itnabadhjatahai ki log sucidetakkarjatehai… Unhewahisahilagtahai..

SUCIDE is not the solution, Its Absolutely WRONG my friends, Taking one's own life can have devastating effects on loved ones and the broader community, and it prevents the possibility of things getting better. If you or someone you know is experiencing thoughts of suicide, it's important to seek professional help as soon as possible. Suicide prevention hotlines and crisis centers are available in many countries and can provide support and resources to help manage suicidal thoughts and feelings. Remember, help is available and there are people who care and want to help you.

Let make the World a beautiful place to life and help ourself as well as other. Preventing suicide involves recognizing the signs of suicidal behavior and taking action to intervene and provide support. Here are some steps you can take to help prevent suicide:

1. Recognize the signs: Be aware of the signs of suicidal behavior, which may include talking about wanting to die or to kill oneself, feeling hopeless or trapped, increased use of alcohol or drugs, withdrawal from friends and family, and changes in mood or behavior.

2. Take it seriously: If you notice any signs of suicidal behavior in someone you know, take it seriously and take action to intervene and provide support.

3. Talk to them: Talk to the person and express your concern. Listen without judgment and provide support and reassurance. Let them know that they are not alone and that help is available.

4. Seek professional help: Encourage the person to seek professional help, such as a therapist, counselor, or psychiatrist. Offer to help them make an appointment and provide transportation if needed.

5. Remove access to means: If the person has access to means of self-harm, such as firearms or medications, remove them from the environment or secure them safely.

6. Follow up: Check in with the person regularly and continue to provide support. Encourage them to follow through with professional help and offer to accompany them to appointments.

Remember, preventing suicide requires everyone's involvement. If you or someone you know is struggling with suicidal thoughts or behavior, seek help immediately. You can call a suicide prevention hotline or seek help from a mental health professional. There is help and hope available.

Dosto, All this feeling are making us more empty, I know IF I say ki shift your focus from all this and do some thing which you actually want to do you may resist and think what the hell gyaannaichaiya but, sach me if you really want to come out of the pain and live a happy life,

I follow 1 simple Rule, & I made it Bold and Clear in my Mind

There Is A Huge Amount Of FREEDOM

That Comes To You, When YOU TAKE

 NOTHING PERSONALLY

Ye jo bimarihainadusre se umeedkarna ki, dusre ki baatdil pe lagane ki, dusrekyasochenga ye sochne ki, dusre k haat me apne life ka remote control dene ki… issbimari se baharniklo, Come out of this dilemma situation,

I have spoken about this thousand times on my speech and I'm making it clear again that : Log kyasochegaissbimari se to dur hoonmai, isliyaaaj jo bhi hu khushhoonmai,

This is YOUR LIFE, Its Your JORNEY, You have to Sit on the Driver Seat, YOU can change the Gear, take a Break orAccelerate in full speed, or be just in Neutral stateChoice is always in your hand, And You have the Full rights to Drive as you want. Accident may happen, so as in life as well, Always remember we can always recover from the injury as well, but giving up once life so easily is not right choice my friend.

Sh*t no 19

<u>Wholeness well-being :</u>

Wholeness & well-being are two inter- related concepts that refer to a state of completeness, balance, & optimal functioning in all aspects of our lives - *physical, emotional, social, &spiritual.*

Wholeness refers to a state of being complete or undivided. In terms of personal well-being, it suggests a state of being fully integrated and balanced in all aspects of our lives, including our physical, mental, emotional, and spiritual health. Wholeness suggests that each aspect of our lives is interconnected and that to be truly healthy and fulfilled, we must strive for balance and integration in all areas.

Well-being, on the other hand, refers to a state of optimal physical, emotional, and social functioning. It encompasses a range of factors that contribute to our overall health and happiness, including physical health, emotional resilience, social support, and a sense of purpose and meaning in life. Well-being is not just the absence of disease or negative symptoms, but rather a state of positive health and vitality.Together, wholeness and well-being represent a holistic approach to heal.

<u>Health</u>is important for many reasons& it's a truth, as it affects all aspects of our lives. It is important for us because it affects every aspect of our lives, including our ability to work, socialize, &enjoy life.Good health allows us to live a happy fulfilling life, free from the limitations that poor health can bring. When we are healthy, we can fully participate in the activities we enjoy, spend time with thepeople we care about, and pursue our goals & ambitions. Good health can also improve our quality of life, increase our longevity, & reduce our risk of developing chronic diseases that can shorten our lives.On the other hand, poor health can have a significant negative impact on our lives. It can limit our ability to work, travel, and enjoy life, and can cause physical, emotional, and financial hardship for ourselves and our families. Poor health can also increase our risk of developing chronic diseases and medical conditions, which can lead to significant medical expenses and decreased quality of life.

Taking care of your health is an ongoing process that requires attention and effort in several areas of your life.

Here are some tips for maintaining good health:

1. Eat a healthy, balanced diet - Include a variety of nutrient-dense foods in your diet, such as fruits, vegetables, whole grains, lean proteins, and healthy fats.

2. Exercise regularly - Aim for at least 30 minutes of moderate-intensity exercise most days of the week. This can include activities such as walking, running, cycling, or strength training.

3. Get enough sleep - Aim for 7-8 hours of sleep per night to help your body recharge and recover.

4. Manage stress - Practice stress management techniques

such as deep breathing, meditation, or yoga to help reduce stress levels and promote relaxation.

5. Stay hydrated - Drink plenty of water throughout the day to help keep your body functioning properly.

6. Avoid harmful habits - Avoid smoking, excessive alcohol consumption, and drug use to help reduce your risk of developing chronic health conditions.

7. Stay up-to-date on preventive health measures - This includes regular check-ups with your doctor, recommended cancer screenings, and vaccinations.

8. Take care of your mental health - Engage in activities that promote positive mental health, such as spending time with loved ones, pursuing hobbies, or seeking professional help if needed.

As per Ayurveda:

Here are some key principles of Ayurveda that can help promote good health:

1. Understanding your dosha - Ayurveda categorizes people into three doshas or body types - Vata, Pitta, and Kapha. Understanding your dominant dosha can help you make dietary and lifestyle choices that are best suited to your unique needs.

2. Eating a balanced diet - Ayurveda recommends eating a variety of fresh, whole foods that are appropriate for your

dosha. It also emphasizes the importance of mindful eating and avoiding overeating.

3. Practicing self-care - Ayurveda places great importance on self-care practices, such as daily massage, meditation, yoga, and other relaxation techniques.

4. Managing stress - Ayurveda recognizes the negative impact of stress on the body and offers several relaxation techniques to help reduce stress levels.

5. Maintaining a healthy digestive system - Ayurveda places great importance on maintaining a healthy digestive system, as it is believed to be the root of good health. This can be achieved through a healthy diet, regular exercise, and stress management.

6. Using natural remedies - Ayurveda uses a range of natural remedies, such as herbs, oils, and other natural substances, to help promote healing and prevent disease.

By incorporating these habits into your daily routine, you can help promote good health and reduce your risk of developing chronic health conditions. Remember, taking care of your health is an ongoing process, so focus on making small, sustainable changes that you can maintain over time.

Sari bimariya mostly start hotihai pet se so taking care of you Gut.

The gut plays a critical role in overall health, as it is responsible for digesting food, absorbing nutrients, and eliminating waste. Here are some tips to improve your gut health:

1. Eat a balanced, whole foods-based diet - A diet rich in fibres, like leafy vegetables, oats whole grains, and lean protein sources can provide the necessary nutrients for a healthy gut, Flax seed, chia seed or sabja seed very good alternative.

2. Incorporate prebiotic and probiotic foods - Prebiotic foods such as garlic, onions, and bananas provide the necessary fuel for healthy gut bacteria, while probiotic foods such as yogurt, kefir, and sauerkraut introduce healthy bacteria into the gut.

3. Avoid processed foods and Stay hydrated - Drinking plenty of water can help promote healthy digestion and regularity Take Chaas also known as salted buttermilk every day in the afternoon.

4. Consider supplements - Certain supplements, such as probiotics or digestive enzymes, may be helpful in promoting a healthy gut. However, it is important to consult with a healthcare professional before beginning any new supplement regimen.

v Amla - Known as Indian gooseberry, is a fruit that

has been used in traditional Ayurvedic medicine for thousands of years due to its numerous health benefits.

Here are some properties of amla:

Rich in vitamin C - An important antioxidant that can help boost the immune system and protect against cellular damage. help reduce inflammation in the body and reduce the risk of chronic disease. May help regulate blood sugar levels, Good for digestive health Promotes healthy skin and hair, improve liver function, some studies suggest that amla may have anti-cancer properties, although more research is needed to fully understand its potential effects. It's also used for improving memory and brain health. The list is goes on for amLA it's also represent Lord Vishnu. Overall, amla is a nutritious and versatile fruit that can be consumed in a variety of forms, including fresh, dried, or as a supplement, it provides several health benefits.

v Khajur – Also known as Dates are a good source of dietary fiber, which can help promote digestive health, regulate blood sugar levels, and lower cholesterol.

Dates contain several important vitamins and minerals, including potassium, magnesium, and vitamin B6, Good source of antioxidants Natural energy booster.

❖ Secret Recipe: During winter or anytime you like,

Take a small pan put 1 tsp cow ghee heat it and sauté some dates for 2 min and add (as per your taste buds) a pinch of black salt, haldi and black pepper powder and have it hot or as per your preference I'm pretty sure that you all will love this recipe for sure

<u>Similarly Taking care of Mental health is a Precedence for us.</u>

Mental health is like a garden that needs tender care and attention to flourish. Just as a garden needs the right conditions to grow, mental health thrives when we nourish it with love, kindness, and self-compassion.

When we tend to our mental health, we create a sanctuary within ourselves - a place of peace, calm, and inner strength. We learn to cultivate resilience and to weather life's storms with grace and equanimity.

Just as a garden is made up of many different elements - soil, plants, water, and sunlight - mental health is a complex interplay of many factors. It is not something that can be achieved overnight, but a lifelong journey of growth and self-discovery.

So let us tend to our mental health with the same care and devotion that we would give to a beautiful garden. Let us water it with love, nourish it with kindness, and watch it bloom and flourish, in all its infinite beauty.

Mental health is not just the absence of mental illness or disorder, but also the presence of positive attributes such as resilience, self-esteem, and a positive outlook on life. Mental health is influenced by a variety of factors, including genetic, environmental, and social factors, as well as life experiences and circumstances.

Mental health issues can range from mild to severe, and can include anxiety, depression, bipolar disorder, schizophrenia, post-traumatic stress disorder (PTSD), and other conditions. It is important to seek professional help if you are experiencing mental health issues, as there are many effective treatments and therapies available.

Coming out of mental health issues can be a challenging and complex process, but there are many effective strategies and resources available that can help. Here are a few steps you can take to start your journey towards recovery:

1. Seek professional help: A mental health professional, such as a therapist or counselor, can provide you with the guidance, support, and resources you need to overcome mental health issues. They can help you develop coping skills, work through difficult emotions, and provide you

with effective treatments and therapies.

2. Build a support system: Having a strong support system can be a critical part of the recovery process. This can include friends, family members, support groups, and mental health professionals. Surrounding yourself with people who understand and care about you can provide you with the emotional support & encouragement you need to move forward.

3. Take care of your physical health: The mind and body are interconnected, and taking care of your physical health can have a positive impact on your mental health. This can include eating a balanced diet, getting regular exercise, and getting enough sleep.

4. Practice self-care: Taking care of yourself is essential to mental health recovery. This can include engaging in activities that you enjoy, such as reading, art, or meditation. It can also involve setting healthy boundaries, learning to say no when necessary, and being kind to yourself.

5. Stay positive: Recovery from mental health issues can take time, and setbacks are a natural part of the process. Try to stay positive and remind yourself that progress is possible, even if it may not always be linear.

Remember that everyone's journey towards mental health recovery is unique, and there is no one-size-fits-all approach. Be patient with yourself, and don't be afraid to reach out for help and support when you need it.

There are a variety of tools and techniques that can be helpful in healing mental health issues. Here are some examples:

1. Cognitive Behavioural Therapy (CBT): CBT is a type of therapy that focuses on changing negative thought patterns and behaviors that may contribute to mental health issues. This can include identifying negative thought patterns and challenging them with more positive and realistic thinking.

2. Mindfulness Meditation: Mindfulness meditation involves paying attention to the present moment without judgment. This practice has been shown to reduce stress, anxiety, and depression.

3. Physical exercise: Regular exercise can help to reduce symptoms of anxiety and depression, as well as improve overall mood and well-being.

4. Art therapy: Art therapy involves using creative expression to explore and process emotions. It can be a helpful tool for those who may have difficulty expressing themselves verbally.

5. Journaling: Writing down thoughts and feelings can be a helpful way to process emotions and gain perspective on difficult situations.

6. Medication: In some cases, medication may be prescribed to help manage symptoms of mental health issues.

7. Support groups: Participating in a support group with

others who have similar experiences can provide a sense of community and reduce feelings of isolation.

8. NLP – Most powerful and Effective Technique:

Neuro-Linguistic Programming (NLP) is a form of therapy that can be used to improve mental health. NLP focuses on the relationship between a person's thoughts, language, and behavior, and how this can impact mental and emotional states. Here are some ways that NLP can be used for mental health:

1. Reframing negative thoughts: NLP can help individuals identify and reframe negative thoughts that may be contributing to mental health issues. This can involve identifying negative language patterns and replacing them with positive affirmations.

2. Anchoring positive emotions: NLP can be used to anchor positive emotions and experiences to specific triggers, such as a certain sound or touch. This can help individuals access positive emotions when they are feeling down or anxious.

3. Changing limiting beliefs: NLP can help individuals identify and change limiting beliefs that may be holding them back from achieving their goals and improving their mental health.

4. Creating new patterns of behavior: NLP can help individuals create new patterns of behavior that can lead to improved mental health. This can involve setting new

goals, creating positive habits, and developing a stronger sense of self.

Being an NLP Expert :

I have studied and worked on various cases Through NLP techniques, individuals can learn to identify and change negative patterns of thinking and behavior, overcome limiting beliefs, and develop a more positive and empowering mindset. Some common NLP techniques include visualization, reframing, and anchoring, which can help individuals to shift their focus and create new, positive associations in their minds.

While NLP can be a powerful tool for personal growth and healing, it is important to work with a trained and qualified NLP practitioner who can guide you through the process and provide personalized support and guidance. With the right guidance and support, NLP can help individuals to overcome personal challenges, improve their relationships, and live a more fulfilled and meaningful life.

Certainly! NLP is a fascinating and dynamic field with numerous potential benefits that can enhance various aspects of our lives. Learning NLP can provide valuable skills that can help us communicate more effectively, better understand and analyze human language, and make more informed decisions.

With the ability to analyze large volumes of data and extract meaningful insights, NLP can help us make sense of the world around us and improve our decision-making capabilities. Additionally, NLP-powered technologies like chatbots and virtual assistants can provide convenient and personalized support for a variety of tasks, such as customer service, information retrieval, and productivity.

By learning NLP, individuals can gain a deeper understanding of human language and its complexities, which can enhance their communication skills and enable them to connect with others more effectively. Ultimately, these skills and knowledge can contribute to a more fulfilling and successful life, where individuals are better equipped to navigate complex challenges and achieve their goals.

IF you really want to change your life do learn NLP friends it's a Game changer tool for a Successful life. I assure you

This is the Precious Treasure of NLP

Change your self From Current State to Desired State

So, in summary, NLP can provide numerous benefits that can enhance various aspects of our lives and contribute to a more fulfilling and successful life.

THE BRAIN is incredibly complex. It is the most complex organ in the human body, with billions of neurons and trillions of connections between them. The brain is responsible for a wide range of functions, including regulating the body's physical processes, controlling movement and sensation, processing sensory information, and enabling complex cognitive processes such as thought, memory, and emotion.

The brain is made up of several distinct regions, each of which is responsible for different functions. These regions include the cortex, which is responsible for consciousness and higher cognitive functions, as well as the brainstem, cerebellum, and other subcortical structures that control basic bodily functions such as breathing and heart rate.

Despite significant advances in neuroscience research, there is still much that is not fully understood about the brain. Researchers continue to study the brain in order to gain a better understanding of its functions, how it develops and changes over time, and how it can be affected by disease, injury, and environmental factors.

While the brain's complexity can make it challenging to understand, it is also what makes it such an incredible and fascinating organ. The brain's ability to learn, adapt, and grow is what allows us to constantly improve and develop as individuals.

It is important to note that not all tools and techniques will work for everyone, and what may work for one person may not work for another. It is important to work with a mental health professional.

NLP SWISH Technique:

NLP offers a variety of techniques for dealing with unwanted or negative memories. One technique that may be helpful is called the "Swish" pattern. Here are the steps for using the Swish pattern:

1. Identify the bad memory that you want to remove.

2. Choose a positive, resourceful image that you want to replace the bad memory with.

3. Imagine the bad memory in front of you, as if it were on a movie screen. See it in full color, with vivid details.

4. Create a small, black-and-white image of the positive image you chose in step 2. Make it small and place it in the bottom left corner of your mental screen.

5. Now, quickly, & vividly visualize the positive image growing in size until it completely replaces the negative image.Make the positive image bright, colorfulwith details.

6. When the positive image completely covers the negative image, make it "swish" away to the top right corner of your mental screen. See it zoom away like a rocket, leaving only the positive image behind.

7. Repeat steps 4-6 several times, each time making the positive image larger and brighter until the bad memory is replaced by the positive image.

This technique can be very effective for some people, but it's important to note that it may not work for everyone. If you're struggling with a bad memory, it may be helpful to work with a qualified NLP practitioner or therapist who can help guide you through the process.

Sh*t no 20

<u>Lost in Finding :</u>

खोजमेंहमतुम्हारीयूंभटकतेरहे
खोज़खुदकेहीहमफिरमिटातेरहे ।।

मनमांझीसाअबढून्ढताहैतुम्हें
डूबकरभीतुम्हेंहमखुदबचातेरहे ।
अंधेरोमेंभीथीसिर्फतुम्हारीतलाश
दीपसाखुदजलेऔरखुदबुझातेरहे ।
खोजमेंहमतुम्हारीयूंभटकतेरहे
खोज़खुदकेहीहमफिरमिटातेरहे ।।

As we are realizing that in the modern world, many people lead very busy lives that can make it difficult to stay connected to oneself. The demands of work, family, and social obligations can leave little time for self-reflection, self-care, and pursuing one's own interests and passions.

When we become so preoccupied with external demands, we can lose touch with our own values, goals, and sense of purpose. We may start to feel like we're just going through the motions of life, without a clear sense of direction or fulfillment.

If you feel like you have lost yourself in the busyness of life, it may be helpful to take a step back and reassess your priorities. Ask yourself what's truly important to you, and whether the activities and commitments in your life align with those priorities.

It may also be helpful to set aside some time each day for self-care and self-reflection. This could involve activities like meditation, journaling, or spending time in nature. Prioritizing activities that bring you joy and fulfillment, rather than just focusing on productivity or meeting external expectations, can help you stay connected to yourself and your values.

Remember, finding oneself is a journey that takes time and effort. It's important to be patient and kind to yourself throughout the process, and to seek support from loved ones or a therapist if needed. With time and effort, it's possible to reconnect with oneself and live a more fulfilling, authentic life.

finding yourself:

Practice mindfulness: Mindfulness is a powerful tool for becoming more present and connected with yourself. It involves paying attention to your thoughts, emotions, and physical sensations in the moment, without judgment or distraction. Mindfulness practices like meditation, deep breathing, or yoga can be helpful in cultivating this awareness.

Explore your values: Take some time to reflect on what values are most important to you. These might include things like honesty, compassion, creativity, or adventure. Once you have identified your values, make an effort to align your actions and decisions with them.

Set boundaries: It's important to set boundaries and prioritize your own needs in order to stay connected with yourself. This might involve saying no to commitments that don't align with your values, taking breaks when you need them, or communicating your needs to others.

Connect with others: While it's important to prioritize your own needs, it's also important to connect with others and build supportive relationships. Surrounding yourself with people who share your values and interests can be a great way to stay connected with yourself.Be kind to yourself: Finally, it's important to be kind and compassionate to yourself throughout the process of self-discovery. Remember that finding yourself is a journey, and there will be ups and downs along the way. Treat yourself with the same kindness and understanding that you would offer to a close friend or loved one.

*Zindagi me hum khud ko to puri tarahsamajhnahi patekabhikabhi, Logo ko hum kyasamajega.*Its really a bitter truth, We are wearing a color glass which is of our childhood experience and the conditioning which we have received since or even before birth, If we are wearing a blue glass we will see the whole world as Blue, Its our fault and we need to remove the glasses which ever we are wearing, to find out truly who you are There is Test in NLP called PIP test – It works wonders to find oneself. Kuch karo yana karo khud ko sahi se pehchan lo zindagiaasanhojayegijeena me.

Part III

The 3 Question

You should ask yourself for the life you are gifted with.

Q1. Calling of Your Soul?

Throughout childhood we are good at many things we grasp everything fast, childhood is often compared to a soft clay because it is a period of rapid growth and development. During childhood, our brains are still developing, and we are constantly learning and absorbing new information from the world around us. This makes us particularly receptive to experiences and influences that can shape our personalities and perspectives. As like other children, I was good at many thing (except dancing singing ha ha ha) I was always wondering ki ye sab to mujheaatahai par what is my Destiny, And truly speaking Thanks to this Q which turned my world upside down and made me happy to where I'm now "What is that I'm meant for, its not to gain success, or earn more money,

"What is my True calling" and after 30 years of hustle I found what is Life for me, It may take less or more time depending on individual.

"Giving a smile on someone's face, helping others and making a positive difference in the world bring peace and fulfillment to me. Sharing my knowledge, skills, and resources with others, I can make a impact and bring joy and positivity to those around me.

Sukoon is the best word for expressing my feelings

Many times it happens in life and that we express our true feeling in our mother tongue as they are much near to our heart.

The meaning of life can differ from person to person and from time to time. So what matters is not the meaning of life in general, but the meaning of life at the particular moment.

The meaning of life can change but will never cease. The fact that most of us live our lives without knowing what we really need to do and what is the purpose/ meaning of our life. Often people admit to having no future, hope, or meaning in life. They keep on complaining constantly about their life.

Although, there is no shortcut to finding meaning in life, Finding meaning in life gives a purpose to live for. It strengthens resilience even in the face of adversity. Therefore, we all should ask ourselves questions once in a while like who we are and what we need to do.

Finding Meaning Is Therapy for Your Soul but don't lose yourself in finding it. What does it mean for something to mean something? As humans, we have a constant need to attach meaning to everything that happens in our lives.

Example: My mom hugs me, that *mean* that she loves me. It's raining heavily means we should have Fried Pakodas, I'm a grown up now Married and have kids that mean I have more responsibility now, I'm looking fat that means I have to eat less or do large size dress shopping. I dint scored good mark means I have to study more or leave the school.

Meaning is the association that we draw between two experiences or events in our minds. X happens, then Y happens, so we assume that *means* X causes Y. Z happens, and we get really bummed out and feel awful, therefore we assume that Z sucks.

Our brains invent meaning the way dogs shit—they do it gleefully and not even realizing that they're ruining the carpet. Our brains invent meaning as a way to explain all the crazy shit that is going on in the world around us. This is important, as it helps us predict and control our lives. But let's be real: Meaning is an *arbitrary* mental construct.

Fifty people watch the exact same event and draw fifty different meanings from that event. That's why there's so much arguing in politics. That's why eyewitnesses are so unreliable in court. That's why your friends are sometimes the biggest assholes—because that meaning you just shared, to them, meant something completely different.

Meaning is not something that exists outside of ourselves. It is not some cosmic universal truth waiting to be discovered. It is not some grand 'eureka' moment that will change our lives forever. Meaning requires action. Meaning is something that we must continually find and nurture. Consistently.

"The Secret to life is meaningless unless you discover it yourself."

— W. Somerset Maugham

Q2. What makes You really happy & Fulfilled ?

What do I need to be happy and fulfilled? Everyone's definition of happiness and fulfillment is different. Think about the things that bring you joy and make you feel content, whether it's spending time with loved ones, pursuing a hobby, or having a fulfilling career. Identify the things that are most important to your personal sense of happiness and make them a priority in your life.

Frankly speaking Exploring new destination unknown land not so famous, tribal places, mountains, lost places, beaches, make me feel aha... trying the local food, something not tasted before makes my whole heart happy and fulfilled.

What you need to be happy and fulfilled is unique to you and may vary at different points in your life. However, here are some common things that can contribute to happiness and fulfillment:

1. Meaningful relationships: Having strong connections with others, such as close friends and family, can provide a sense of belonging and support that is essential to happiness and fulfillment.

2. Purposeful work: Having work that is meaningful and aligned with your values and interests can give you a sense of purpose and satisfaction. This can include volunteer work or a career that you find fulfilling.

3. Personal growth: Engaging in activities that challenge you and allow you to develop new skills or knowledge can help you feel a sense of progress and accomplishment.

4. Positive mindset: Cultivating a positive mindset and focusing on gratitude and optimism can help you feel happier and more fulfilled.

5. Physical and emotional well-being: Taking care of your physical and emotional health through regular exercise, healthy eating, and self-care can help you feel happier and more energized.

6. Pursuing passions and interests: Making time for activities that you enjoy and that bring you pleasure can help you feel happier and more fulfilled.

Remember that everyone's path to happiness and fulfilment is unique, and what works for one person may not work for another. Take time to reflect on your own values, interests, and needs, and make choices that align with your personal goals and priorities.

Sometimes past traumatic experiences can continue to affect us for years, causing recurring memories and even leading to specific fears or phobias. It can be challenging to move past these experiences, but it's important to work on processing and overcoming them in order to live a fulfilling life free from the weight of the past.

NLP technique called "the fast phobia cure," which is sometimes also referred to as the "Visual-Kinesthetic Dissociation" (VKD) technique. This technique can be used to help individuals overcome phobias and other negative memories or experiences.

The basic steps of the fast phobia cure technique are:

1. Identify the negative memory or experience that you want to address.
2. Visualize the experience as if you are watching it on a TV screen, with yourself as the actor in the scene.
3. As you watch the scene, notice the feelings and sensations that arise in your body.
4. Pause the scene at the point where the negative feelings are at their peak.
5. Begin to dissociate from the scene by making the TV

screen smaller and pushing it away from you, or imagining a remote control that can turn the scene to black and white, turn down the sound, or change the channel.

6. As you dissociate from the scene, notice the negative feelings and sensations becoming weaker and less intense.

7. When the negative feelings are at their weakest, bring the TV screen back to its normal size and color, and watch the scene play out to a positive conclusion.

By repeating this technique a few times, you can often reduce the negative emotional impact of the memory or experience. However, it's important to note that this technique may not be appropriate or effective for everyone, and it's always a good idea to seek the help of a trained NLP practitioner or mental health professional if you're struggling with a traumatic or difficult experience.

Hobbies

Hobbies are activities that we engage in for pleasure and enjoyment, outside of our regular work or daily responsibilities. Hobbies can be a great way to relax, reduce stress, and explore new interests.

The best advice I can give you to be creative and happy "Dedicate some time on your hobbies or what you actually love to do".

If you don't have any hobby that means you have never explored enough in life, find what you really like to do in your free time or take out time from your busy schedule for what you love to do. To make it simpler for you guys, will try to list it down few hobbies, and find what you actually love to do, it may be something apart from it. You need to explore more...

There are many types of hobbies that people enjoy. Here are some examples:

1. Creative hobbies: Examples include painting, drawing, sculpting, pottery, knitting, crocheting, sewing, embroidery, and photography.

2. Sports and outdoor hobbies: Examples include hiking, running, cycling, swimming, surfing, skiing, snowboarding, golf, tennis, basketball, football, soccer, and camping.

3. Music and performing arts hobbies: Examples include singing, playing an instrument, dancing, acting, and theatre.

4. Cooking and baking hobbies: Examples include experimenting with different recipes, baking desserts, and cooking new dishes.

5. Collecting hobbies: Examples include collecting stamps, coins, vinyl records, vintage items, or other memorabilia.

6. Gaming hobbies: Examples include video games, board games, card games, and puzzles.

7. Reading and writing hobbies: Examples include reading

books, writing stories, poetry, Reading and writing hobbies: Examples include reading books, writing stories, poetry, or journals.

7. Traveling and exploring hobbies: Examples include exploring new places, visiting museums and art galleries, and trying out different cuisines.

8. Gardening: Many people enjoy planting and caring for their own gardens, whether it's a small herb garden or a large vegetable plot.

9. Home improvement: DIY projects, such as painting, building furniture, or remodeling a room, can be a satisfying way to improve one's home.

10. Volunteer work: Giving back to the community by volunteering for a cause or organization can be a fulfilling hobby for many.

11. Meditation and mindfulness: Some people find relaxation and stress relief through practices such as meditation, yoga, or tai chi.

12. Language learning: Studying a new language can be a challenging and rewarding hobby that can open new opportunities for travel and cultural experiences.

13. Fishing: For those who enjoy the outdoors and being by the water, fishing can be a calming and enjoyable pastime.

14. Board game design: Some people enjoy creating their own board games, playtesting and refining the rules and gameplay.

15. Astronomy: Studying the stars and the universe can be a fascinating hobby that requires only a telescope and a clear night sky.

16. Geocaching: This modern-day treasure hunt involves using GPS coordinates to find hidden caches or containers that have been placed around the world.

17. Genealogy: Tracing one's family tree and learning about ancestors can be a rewarding hobby that connects people to their heritage and history.

18. Animal Love, Pet care, Pet ownership: Many people enjoy having pets and caring for their animals, whether it's a dog, cat, bird, fish, or any other type of animal. Animal rescue and adoption: Some animal lovers dedicate their time and resources to rescuing and fostering animals in need, and helping them find loving homes. One friend of mine he loves to catch snakes and then he goes to jungle and leave them there safe. I have the one who loves dogs and cats and she is busy whole day talking to them and taking care for them.

"I love to Play with Colors, I have a passion for colors and design, and I've used it to create a unique and personalized space in my home. I've personally designed each wall in a unique style, each wall has its own story to tell. I also enjoy painting on canvas, and it's been a true blessing to have people appreciate my art. I'm grateful for the opportunity to share my creativity with others and bring joy through my art." There is a painting which I painted, photo has been shared in starting of the book Bappa, Ganpati Ji.

It will look like black and whiteas per printing colors but the true colors are really magical, If you wish to see the real paintingYou can visit my Insta handle @alayna_sonar

I enjoy exploring my creativity and experimenting with different materials and techniques to make unique and personal pieces. The best part about DIY is that there are always new skills to learn and new projects to try. It's a hobby that allows me to express myself and also make a positive impact on the environment by repurposing items and reducing waste. All in all, DIY and creativity are a huge part of my life and bring me so much happiness and fulfillment."

What's Yours Hobbies my dear:_______________________________

____

Exploring new hobbies and interests can be a wonderful and exciting experience! Trying something new can be a great way to challenge yourself, expand your horizons, and discover new passions.

Whether it's learning a new language, taking up a new sport, or picking up a musical instrument, trying something new can be a fulfilling and enriching experience. It can also be a great way to meet new people, learn new skills, and gain a fresh perspective on life.

So, if you're looking for a new hobby, don't be afraid to step out of your comfort zone and try something new. You never know what you might discover and the feeling of accomplishment and growth that comes from learning a new skill or pursuing a new interest can be truly awesome!

Q3.What Legacy do I want to leave behind?

I think it's the most heart storming Question for all, think about the impact you want to have on the world and or even the few people around you. Consider what you want to be remembered for, and what kind of mark you want to make on the world. Consider the positive impact that you would like to have on others and the world around you. This can include things like helping others, making a difference in your community, or leaving the world a better place than you found it.

Think about the skills, resources, and opportunities that you have to make a positive impact. This can include volunteer work, philanthropy, or even the way you interact with others on a daily basis. What values do you want to instill in others? Consider the values that are most important to you, such as compassion, kindness, or generosity. Think about ways that you can model these values and inspire others to live by them as well.

Remember that your legacy is not just about the impact that you make on the world, but also the impact that you make on the people around you. By living a life that aligns with your values and priorities, you can inspire others to do the same and leave a lasting impact on the world.

Write down your vision for your legacy and plan for how you can work towards it. It doesn't mean that You have to become Mahatma Gandhi, Mother Terrace, Nichola Tesla or Einstein, You can be you and can be remembered as you if you make someone smile or help with what you have.

Here I will share a story of my life : We were a middle class family, My father was a service man, who is no more with us it's been 10 yrs. But people still remember him as the most kind and happy person they ever met.

Wo jissabhimiltethayaatejate wo sabkonamsteboltethay ek pyarisi smile k sath, Papa ki salary bahut kamthi as I already mention we were staying in chawl, to humare pass ghumne ko yaphirbaharkhane k paisa naihotethayitna, But sachbolukabiiskaafsosnai hu ana kabi kami mehsus ki, kyo ki Paapahumeharweakend pe bahar le jatethay, Chawl k sab bachaa ko leke pass wali ground pe cricket khilatethayaur golakhilatethaysabko, to kabi airport k pass wali garden se plane dikhatethay aur jhoolajhulatethay, to kabi double decker bus me Juhu beach le jatethay aur waha pe apnehato se ghar pe hi pani-puri ya sandwich bana k le jate aur hum sunset k sath wo nazar enjoy kartethay, That were the most beautiful sunsets of my life, That's the reason beaches are my 2nd home sukoonmiltahaiwaha jo kahinaimiltasamandar ki lehro ki awaz sun k, aisalagtahai papa bularahehai beta, aur aage mat jaogehrahaipaniwanhasambhal k..

I still got emotional while writing this line felt as if he was sitting beside me.

All I want you to feel what legacy you want to leave behind once you are no more and people would remember you for that. Do share your feelings, trust me you will feel happy while doing this task.

Legacy that I wanted to leave behind:

____

____

____

____

If you don't have any such thoughtin your mind what to do then

I would like to suggest something which I do.

Just plant trees every year on your Birth day &Nourish them with your love and care.

This can be counted as your legacy because you did something wonderful for the Mother Earth and for our environment :)

#The 3 Formulas

1. <u>Trust yourself - You are enough</u>

"Trust in yourself, believe that your voice matters,

And know that your words are good enough

To shout out loud your thoughts"

Trusting yourself is about having faith in your abilities, values, and intuition. It means learning to listen to your inner voice, even when it goes against the opinions of others. When you trust yourself, you're better equipped to handle challenges, take risks, and pursue your dreams. You're less likely to get stuck in indecision or self-doubt because you know that you have what it takes to succeed. Cultivating self-trust takes time and practice, but it's worth it. By developing a strong sense of self-worth and confidence, you can create a fulfilling life that aligns with your true self. So trust yourself, be true to yourself, and let your light shine.

I remember that days, I had a really tough time when I was feeling helpless and unworthy. I remember how difficult it was to get through each day and how much it felt like a struggle against the wind to find self.

But looking back on that time, I can also see how much I've grown and learned since then. I've developed a greater sense of compassion and empathy for myself and others who may be going through similar struggles. I've also learned how to cope with difficult emotions and to recognize my own resilience and inner strength.

Although that period of my life was challenging, I can reframe it as a time of growth and transformation. I am stronger and more resilient now because of what I went through, and I know that I have the ability to overcome any future challenges that come my way.

The only thought made me where I'm now Trust in myself and having the feeling that I'm Enough. I have all what I need, I'm not less than anyone in this word, I'm ME MYSELF

Now, every day I wake up with the conviction that I am destined for greatness. The thought of being able to make a positive impact on the world fills me with motivation and excitement. I know that I have the power within me to turn my dreams into reality. I refuse to let self-doubt or fear hold me back from reaching my full potential.

I embrace my individuality and understand that my unique qualities are what make me special. I am proud of who I am and confident in my abilities. I am constantly learning and growing, and I know that there is no limit to what I can achieve.

When faced with obstacles or setbacks, I remain steadfast in my belief that I will succeed. I channel my inner strength and resilience to persevere through challenges, knowing that each hurdle I overcome brings me one step closer to my goals.

In short, I am a force to be reckoned with. I trust in myself, I am enough, and I am ready to take on the world with all the passion and determination I possess.

Here's a tip my friend, Just wake up in the Morning and play some dhin-chak music and shout out loud as if your soul is listening and the world is waiting for you…

1. **"I am enough just as I am."**

2. **"I am capable of achieving great things."**

3. **"I am strong, resilient, & capable of overcoming**

   any challenges in my life."

4. **"I have the power within me to create the life I want."**

5. **"I am worthy of love, respect, and success."**

6. **"I trust myself to make the right decisions for my life."**

7. **"I am confident in my abilities and believe in myself."**

8. **"I have everything I need within me to succeed."**

9. **"I am deserving of happiness and fulfillment."**

10. "I embrace my flaws and imperfections; they make me unique and beautiful."

2. <u>STOP – Ignore.com</u>

"Freeing yourself by Saying STOP to Negative Self-Talk and IGNORING.COM to the toxic vibes around You.

(Choose your environment wisely) By applying this formula you are likely to opening a window to a fresh breeze. It's important to recognize and stop the harm you inflict on yourself with negative self-talk. Similarly, don't let external negativity drag you down. Protect your energy and focus on positive thoughts and uplifting vibes. By nurturing a positive mindset, you'll experience a newfound sense of empowerment and inner peace. Embrace the beauty of positivity and let it transform your life."

"Embracing your emotions is like giving yourself an elixir of life. Don't suppress your feelings, learn to understand them. Instead of forcing positivity, transform negativity into something nourishing for your soul. With this mindset shift, you can elevate your well-being and feel the beauty of emotional transformation."

Stop negative self-talk and also pull yourself out from negative talking & poor minded people or environment :

Both can be challenging, but with consistent effort & practice, it is possible. Here are some strategies you can use:

1. Recognize the negative self-talk: Start by becoming aware of your negative self-talk. Notice when you're engaging in self-criticism and try to identify the specific thoughts and beliefs that underlie them.

2. Challenge the negative thoughts: Once you recognize your negative self-talk, challenge those thoughts. Ask yourself if they're based on facts or assumptions. Try to reframe those thoughts in a more positive and compassionate way.

3. Practice self-compassion: Be kind and gentle with yourself. Acknowledge your strengths and accept your flaws. Treat yourself as you would treat a friend who is going through a difficult time.

4. Focus on the present: Negative self-talk is often rooted in the past or future. Try to stay focused on the present moment and engage in activities that bring you joy and fulfillment.

5. Surround yourself with positivity: Surround yourself with

positive people, read positive books, listen to uplifting music, and watch inspiring videos. Fill your life with positivity, and it will help you combat negative self-talk.

Replace negative self Talk

Replacing negative self-talk with positive self-talk is an effective way to promote self-acceptance, boost self-esteem, and improve mental well-being. Here are some examples of positive self-talk that you can use are as follows :

1. Instead of saying "I'm not good enough", say "I am capable and competent in my own way."

2. Instead of saying "I always mess things up", say "I am learning and growing from my mistakes."

3. Instead of saying "I can't do this", say "I will try my best and see what happens."

4. Instead of saying "I'm so stupid", say "I am intelligent and have unique strengths and talents."

5. Instead of saying "I'm a failure", say "I am worthy and valuable regardless of my mistakes or failures."

6. Instead of saying "I'm so awkward and weird", say "I am unique and special, and that makes me interesting."

7. Instead of saying "I'm so fat and ugly", say "I am beautiful and valuable just the way I am."

8. Instead of saying "I'm so lazy and unproductive", say "I am taking a break to recharge and will get back to work soon."

9. Instead of saying "I'm unlucky", say "I am grateful for the blessings in my life & looking forward for more good things to come in my life."

10. Instead of saying "I'm so overwhelmed and stressed", say "I am capable of managing my stress & taking care of myself."

Remember, positive self-talk is a skill that can be developed with practice. The more you use positive self-talk, the more natural andautomatic it will become, leading to a more positive and optimistic outlook on life.

We have heard such dialogues/ muhavras from society that :

"Jitnichaadar ho utne hi pair failao" - This muhavra means that one should limit their actions and expectations based on the available

resources or capacity. It is used to indicate the importance of being practical and realistic in one's approach.

Why should we restrict our desire, rather we can increase the Length of the chadar by working more passionately.

*"**Laalach buri balahai** "* - This muhavra means that greed is a bad thing. It is used to indicate the negative consequences of being too greedy or desirous.*Why is that wanting more is greediness? It's your desire, Every individual should have big dreams…*

*"**Jiskokuchnahichahiye, usko sab kuchmiltahai"*** - This muhavra means that those who do not have excessive desires tend to receive everything. It is used to indicate that those who are content with what they have tend to be more satisfied and fulfilled.

*It's a total *** according to my thought. Agar aapChahogenahi to milegakaisa ???Mangogenaitokoidegakaisa???*

*"**Akalmand ko ishara hi kafihotahai"*** - This muhavra means that intelligent people can understand something just by a sign or hint. It is used to indicate the power intelligence & quickcomprehension

Every individual is different if he/she doesn't know the language of your signs that doesn't mean they are dumb. Some people need clarification in words to put on.

*"**Nekikardariyameindaal"*** - This muhavra means that one should do good deeds without expecting anything in return. It is used to indicate that doing good is its own reward, and one should not be motivated by personal gain.*Why? I'm asking Why… If you put your heart and soul into something, why should we not expect. Expecting is upright but hurting yourself, going into a negative thought pattern after not receiving is not at all a good idea.*

"Jitniunchai par baithoge, utnizor se girnahoga" - This muhavra means that the higher one climbs, the harder they fall. It is used to indicate the potential risks and consequences of success and the importance of maintaining balance and perspective.

Kyobahi... aisakyosochte ho. Yea bhi to sochsakte ho... "More you climb the higher is the chance to fly high ... I believe Sky is not the only limit it's beyond the Galaxy... The point is that you have to be cautious because "With great power comes great responsibility".

"By sharing my thoughts with you, I hope to create a positive impact on your life and empower you to become the best version of yourself.

It's okay if we have different perspectives, as we can learn from each other and grow together. Let's focus on thinking positively and nurturing a mindset that promotes success and fulfillment in all areas of our lives."

As Chanakya quoted beautifully:

*Your **THOUGHTS**will influence your **WORDS**,*

*Which determines your **ACTION**, Over time*

*Your Action will define Your **HABITS***

And those habit regardless of good or bad,

*Determines your **CHARACTER***

*And Finally, Your Character determines Your **DESTINY***

So the conclusion is clear that :

"Choosing your Destiny is in your hands"

And by Altering your thoughts You definitely CAN..

3. Give best shot Every time

Life is a journey, with ups and downs, A winding road that can take us to different towns. Sometimes the path is smooth and clear, Other times, it's rough and filled with fear.But with every twist and every turn, We learn and grow, and we start to discern The beauty in the struggle, the lessons in the pain, The silver lining that is not in vain.For every peak, there's a valley below, Every sunrise follows a sunset's glow. The highs and lows, the joys and tears, Are what make the journey of life so dear.

They teach us to cherish the moments of bliss and appreciate the people we love and miss. They show us our strength, our courage, our grace, and how we can find our way in life's maze.

So when the road gets bumpy and steep, Remember that the journey is not just a leap, It's a process of growth, of learning, of change, And in the end, it's the journey that remains.

Here's An inspiring story is that of Anne Frank

Anne was a Jewish teenager living in Amsterdam during World War II when she and her family went into hiding to escape the Nazi persecution of Jewish people. While in hiding, Anne kept a diary in which she documented her thoughts, feelings, and experiences.

Tragically, Anne and her family were eventually discovered and taken to a concentration camp where Anne died at the age of 15. However, her diary was discovered and published, becoming a worldwide sensation and a poignant reminder of the horrors of the Holocaust.Anne's story is one of resilience, hope, and the power of the written word. Despite the unspeakable suffering and fear that she and her family faced, Anne continued to find beauty and meaning in the world around her. Her diary not only provides a window into the experiences of Jewish people during the

Holocaust, but also serves as a powerful testament to the human spirit and the importance of personal expression and storytelling.

Anne's story reminds us of the importance of bearing witness to the world around us, even in the most difficult of circumstances. It also teaches us the power of hope and resilience, even in the face of unimaginable adversity.

Here's Another inspiring & meaningful story of Nelson Mandela

One of the most inspiring and meaningful stories of overcoming life hurdles is that of Nelson Mandela. Mandela was a South African anti-apartheid revolutionary who spent 27 years in prison for his activism. During his imprisonment, he faced unimaginable hardship and adversity, but he refused to give up his fight for justice and equality.After being released from prison, Mandela continued to work for the betterment of his country and was eventually elected as the first black president of South Africa in 1994. He worked tirelessly to bring an end to apartheid and to promote reconciliation and peace between different racial groups in the country.

Mandela's story is not just one of overcoming personal adversity, but also of fighting for a greater cause and inspiring others to do the same. He believed in the power of forgiveness and reconciliation, and his leadership and advocacy helped to bring about significant social and political change in South Africa.

What makes Mandela's story particularly meaningful, and inspiring is that he did not seek revenge or retribution for the injustices that he and his people had suffered. Instead, he chose to work towards a peaceful and just society, one that embraced the diversity and humanity of all its citizens.

Mandela's life and legacy remind us that even in the face of the most extreme injustice and adversity, we can choose to respond with compassion, forgiveness, and a commitment to social change. His story is a testament to the power of resilience, courage, and hope in the face of great challenges.

Another inspiring example is that of J.K. Rowling,

"When life gives you lemons, make lemonade" is a common saying that encourages us to make the best of a bad situation. This phrase is often used to describe the attitude of turning a negative situation into something positive or productive.

One real-life example of this is the story of J.K. Rowling, the author of the Harry Potter series. Before she became a successful writer, Rowling faced significant setbacks and challenges in her life. She was a single mother struggling to make ends meet, and her first book was rejected by multiple publishers before finally being accepted.

Instead of giving up on her dream of becoming a writer, Rowling used her setbacks as motivation to work harder and persevere. She continued to write and submit her work, eventually finding success with the HarryPotter series, which became worldwide phenomenon.

Rowling's story is a great example of making the best of a bad situation. She could have easily given up after being rejected by so many publishers, but instead, she used the rejection as an opportunity to improve her writing and keep trying. She also used her own struggles as a single mother as inspiration for the character of Harry Potter, who also faced significant challenges and setbacks but continued to fight for what was right.

By taking a difficult situation and turning it into something positive, Rowling was able to achieve her dreams and inspire millions of readers around the world. Her story shows us that even in the face of significant setbacks and challenges, we can choose to be resilient and keep striving towards our goals, ultimately achieving great success and making a positive impact on the world.

These stories remind us that life hurdles are a part of the journey, but they do not have to define us. With resilience, determination, and a strong sense of purpose, we can overcome even the toughest of challenges and emerge stronger and more inspired than ever before. They show us that no matter what obstacles we may face, we can choose to keep going and never give up on our dreams.

<u>Love the Process don't chase for the End results</u>

Love the process of your work, & cherish every task, For it's in the journey of your life, That true fulfillment lasts.With each step that you take, And each moment that you give, You're building your own path, And finding your own way to live.Don't focus on the end result, Or the prize that you seek to win, For the joy is in the effort, And the journey that lies within.Take pleasure in each challenge, And learn from every mistake, For they are the stepping stones, That lead to the life you'll make.

So love the process of your work, And savor every task, For it's in the doing that you'll find, The happiness that will last."The stars are the jewels of the night sky, and they twinkle like theeyes of angels, reminding us that even in the darkness, there isbeauty and light to be found."We often become so focused onachieving our goals and reaching our desired outcomes that weforget about the journey that leads us there. But the journey, the process, the ups and downs, the learning experiences, and the hard work that we put in along the way, are what give meaning to our lives. It is through the journey that we grow and become better versions of ourselves. It is where we find our purpose, learn valuable lessons, &make unforgettable memories.

When we embrace the process and see the beauty in the journey, it can change the way we approach everything in life. It allows us to enjoy the present moment and appreciate the small things that we often take for granted. It helps us to develop patience, resilience, and a growth mindset. It teaches us that success is not just about the outcome, but also about the effort, and the lessons that we learn along the way.

So the next time you're working towards a goal or a dream, remember that the journey is just as important as the destination. Take your time, enjoy the ride, and learn from every experience. Don't let the fear of failure or the desire for instant gratification rob you of the joy that can be found in the process. We often chase after the result, And forget about the journey we're on, But it's in the process of our work, That we truly find where we belong. The destination may be our goal, But the road we take to get there, Is filled with lessons and stories, That enrich and inspire and prepare. Don't rush to the end too quickly, Or overlook the steps in between, For it's in the journey of your life, That the real magic can be seen. Embrace the twists and turns, And find joy in every mile, For it's the path that you're walking, That makes your story worth the while. So let go of the end result, And relish in the work you do, For it's the process of your journey, That will ultimately see you through.

One thing I have understood that Success is not a destination, That we one day arrive at, It's a journey that we undertake, And a path that we grow into at that. It's not just about the finish line, Or the prize that we hope to gain, It's about the effort that we put in, And the progress that we make along the way.

Success is not something that's given, or a blessing that falls from above, It's a reward that we earn through hard work, And the resilience that comes from love. So let us not get caught up in the end goal, Or the dreams that we wish to achieve, let us focus on the journey we take, & the character that we choose to leave. For success is not a destination, it's a process that we undergo, & the moments we spend on the journey, Are the moments that help us grow.

Love the process &journey of your life, Embrace each step and all the strife, Don't get caught up in what's to come, Or chase something from something, then some.Enjoy the moments that life brings, The simple joys and little things, Take time to appreciate the present, And all the blessings that you're sent.Don't rush to the end, don't be in a hurry, For there is much to see and much to worry, It's in the process that we learn and grow, And our true selves begin to show.

So love the process and journey of your life, Take each step with grace and without strife, And you'll find that the destination will come, When you're enjoying the journey and having fun.

#The 3 Fundas

As Today's life

1.   <u>Screenshots</u>

You may be wondering why this term is in this part of the book, and how does it is a fundas of life…

We all may have lots and lots of screenshot saved in our cell phones, am I right or am I right…(If it's not means you are exceptional) In real life, screenshots have become an increasingly common way for people to capture and share their experiences with others. Whether it's capturing a funny meme, a poignant moment from a video call, or a helpful error message from a technical support team, screenshots have become an integral part of our digital communication. Screenshots can also be a valuable tool for documentation and record-keeping.

Life can be compared to a screenshot in the sense that it captures a single moment in time, freezing it in a digital image that can be revisited and reflected upon. Just as a screenshot captures a momentary glimpse of reality, our experiences and memories of life are also fleeting and constantly changing.

Like a screenshot, our memories of life are influenced by the context in which we find ourselves, and are filtered through our own biases and interpretations. The moments we capture in a screenshot may hold different meanings for different people, just as our experiences of life may be interpreted and understood in different ways.

Furthermore, just as a screenshot can be altered or manipulated, our memories and perceptions of life can also be shaped by our own biases, beliefs, and perspectives. The accuracy and authenticity of a screenshot may be called into question, just as our own memories and perceptions of life may be subject to distortions and misrepresentations.

Overall, life can be compared to a screenshot in that it represents a momentary glimpse of reality that is subject to interpretation, alteration, and manipulation. Yet, just as a screenshot can hold valuable information and insights, our experiences and memories of life can offer us important lessons and reflections that can shape our understanding of ourselves and the world around us.

Additionally,

Life can also be compared to a screenshot in terms of the choices we make. Just as we have the power to choose what we capture in a screenshot, we also have the power to choose the experiences and moments we want to hold onto in our memories of life.

The moments we choose to capture in a screenshot may reflect our interests, values, and priorities, just as the experiences we choose to hold onto in our memories of life may reflect the things that are most important to us.

Furthermore, just as a screenshot captures a single moment in time, our lives are made up of a series of interconnected moments that together form a larger narrative. Each screenshot we take represents a piece of a larger puzzle, just as each experience and memory we hold onto forms a part of our personal story.

The moments we capture in a screenshot may bring us joy, sadness, or a range of other emotions, just as our memories of life may evoke a range of feelings and reflections.

Overall, life can be seen as a series of interconnected moments that together form a larger narrative, much like a screenshot captures a single moment that contributes to a larger picture. By choosing to capture and hold onto certain experiences and memories, we can shape the story of our lives and reflect on the things that are most important to us.

"Just as our collection of screenshots can become cluttered and difficult to manage, our memories of life can also become overwhelming and difficult to navigate. Over time, we may accumulate a vast collection of memories, both positive and negative, that can be difficult to organize &process. Therefore, like our collection of screenshots, it is important to periodically review our memories of life and reflect on their significance. We can ask ourselves questions such as: Why do I hold onto this memory? What does this memory mean to me? How has this memory influenced my life?

By taking the time to reflect on our memories of life, we can gain a deeper understanding of ourselves and our personal narrative. We can also identify patterns or themes in our memories that can offer valuable insights into our values, priorities, and experiences.Just as it is important to delete screenshots that are no longer needed or relevant, it is also important to let go of memories that no longer serve us. This does not mean that we should forget or ignore our past, but rather that we should release any negative or harmful memories that are holding us back from living a fulfilling life.

Overall, by periodically reviewing our collection of screenshots and our memories of life, we can better manage and organize our experiences and insights. This can help us to live a more intentional and meaningful life, and to focus on the memories and experiences that truly matter to us.

Our lives are like a gallery of pictures,
A collection of moments that we treasure.
Memories captured, some bright and some dim,
A gallery that grows, with every single whim.

Just like screenshots on our phones,
Our memories can pile up and grow.
But it's important to declutter, to let go of the old,
And keep only what truly touches our soul.

For every screenshot that we take,
We must decide what's worth the keep.
The same with our memories, we must decide,
Which ones we want to cherish and which to release.

Letting go doesn't mean we forget,
Or ignore the moments that we've had.
It simply means we make space,
For the memories that make us glad.

So let us declutter our gallery of life,
And keep only the memories that truly shine.
For in doing so, we make room for more,
And our gallery grows even more divine.

To be continued in 2nd part of the book...

I'm delighted to have had the opportunity to share my insights and experiences with you in this book. I hope that the stories, reflections, and practical advice I've provided have been helpful and inspiring to you.

As we look forward to the second part of the book, I encourage you to take some time to reflect on what you've learned so far and consider how you can implement these lessons in your own life. Remember that personal growth and transformation take time, effort, and commitment, so don't be afraid to start small and build from there.

I'm always eager to hear from my readers, so please don't hesitate to share your feedback with me. Your thoughts and opinions are valuable to me, and I'm grateful for any insights or suggestions you may have.

In conclusion, I hope that this book has provided you with a glimpse into my journey as a purposepreneur and empowered you with the knowledge, tools, and strategies you need to unlock your full potential and achieve your soul goals. Thank you for joining me on this journey, and I look forward to exploring deeper with you in the second part of the book.

About the Author

Alayna Sonar

She is a charismatic and powerful personality who exudes purpose and dedication in all aspects of her life. Her unwavering commitment to helping others achieve self-sufficiency and live fulfilling lives is nothing short of inspiring. As a philanthropist, Alayna uses resources, and influence to promote the well-being of others and improve the quality of life in society andas a purposepreneuris a natural-born leader who empowers people with her wealth of knowledge, tools, and strategies to overcome obstacles & reach their goals. And focus on sustainability, social responsibility, ethical practices, or other values that align with her vision for a better future and making a positive impact on society and the environment.

Alayna's holistic approach to healing and transformation sets her apart as a truly remarkable individual. Her deep understanding of spiritual wisdom, practical solutions, tools, and techniques makes her an invaluable asset to those seeking to unlock their potential and create the life they desire.

Alayna's infectious enthusiasm and positive energy light up any room she enters, leaving a lasting impression on all who meets her.

She has created a powerful platform to share her empowering perspectives and insights with the world. Her magical and unwavering passion for helping others leaves a trail of inspired individuals wherever she goes. If you're looking to tap into your full potential and live a life of abundance and fulfillment, Alayna's powerful and enthralling personality will surly help you achieve your soul goals and set you on the path to success.

@alayna_sonar

@alayna_sonar

Alaynasofficial@gmail.com

520 741

808 897

Signing Off:

Alayna Sonar

Concluding words:

Achieving a great life may seem difficult, and many people settle for less because of life's circumstances, However, if you take the time to understand and apply the knowledge you've gained from this book, and approach your goals with determination, positivity, and tenacity, you can avoid being one of those people. With each small step you take, you'll create an unstoppable momentum that brings you closer to the life you've always wanted.

It's important to remember that every challenge and failure comes with a lesson. Instead of seeing your failures as an endpoint, view them as a twist in your path towards greatness. When you put your heart and soul into something and it doesn't work out, it's not a complete failure. Instead, consider it a sign from the Universe that it wasn't the right thing for you at that moment. Something better is on its way, so don't give up. Keep moving forward.

It's important to trust your intuition and listen to your inner voice when it comes to your relationships and time management. If your gut tells you that a relationship is toxic or that you're wasting your time on something, pay attention and take action. It's essential to set and respect personal boundaries and communicate them to others as well. If something doesn't feel right, it probably isn't, and if something feels amazing and aligned with your values, it's worth pursuing.

By letting go of fear and having faith, your life can shift from ordinary to extraordinary. When you fully commit to your personal growth and strive to live your life with purpose, you'll naturally connect with your higher purpose. Trust the journey, even when it gets challenging, because every experience is an opportunity for growth and learning. So keep pushing forward with determination and a positive attitude, and watch as your life transforms.

The foundation for creating an exciting and fulfilling life starts with loving & Trusting yourself. When you focus on building and maintaining a high vibration, you'll attract more positive experiences and opportunities into your life. Even if it takes time to achieve your dreams, your happy feelings will make the journey feel good along the way. After all, isn't living a life that feels good the ultimate goal?

I can promise you that dedicating yourself to loving and respecting yourself will lead you to incredible achievements. While the path may not always be easy, and sacrifices may need to be made, the end result will be worth it. Remember that you have the power to create the life you want, and it all starts with taking care of yourself and focusing on what brings you joy and fulfilment in your life do what makes you smile. So, I encourage you to take the necessary steps to love and care for yourself, and to never give up on your dreams. With hard work, determination, and a positive attitude, you can achieve greatness and live the life you've always envisioned. The power is in your hands.

-----------------------8080808008080808080808---------------------------

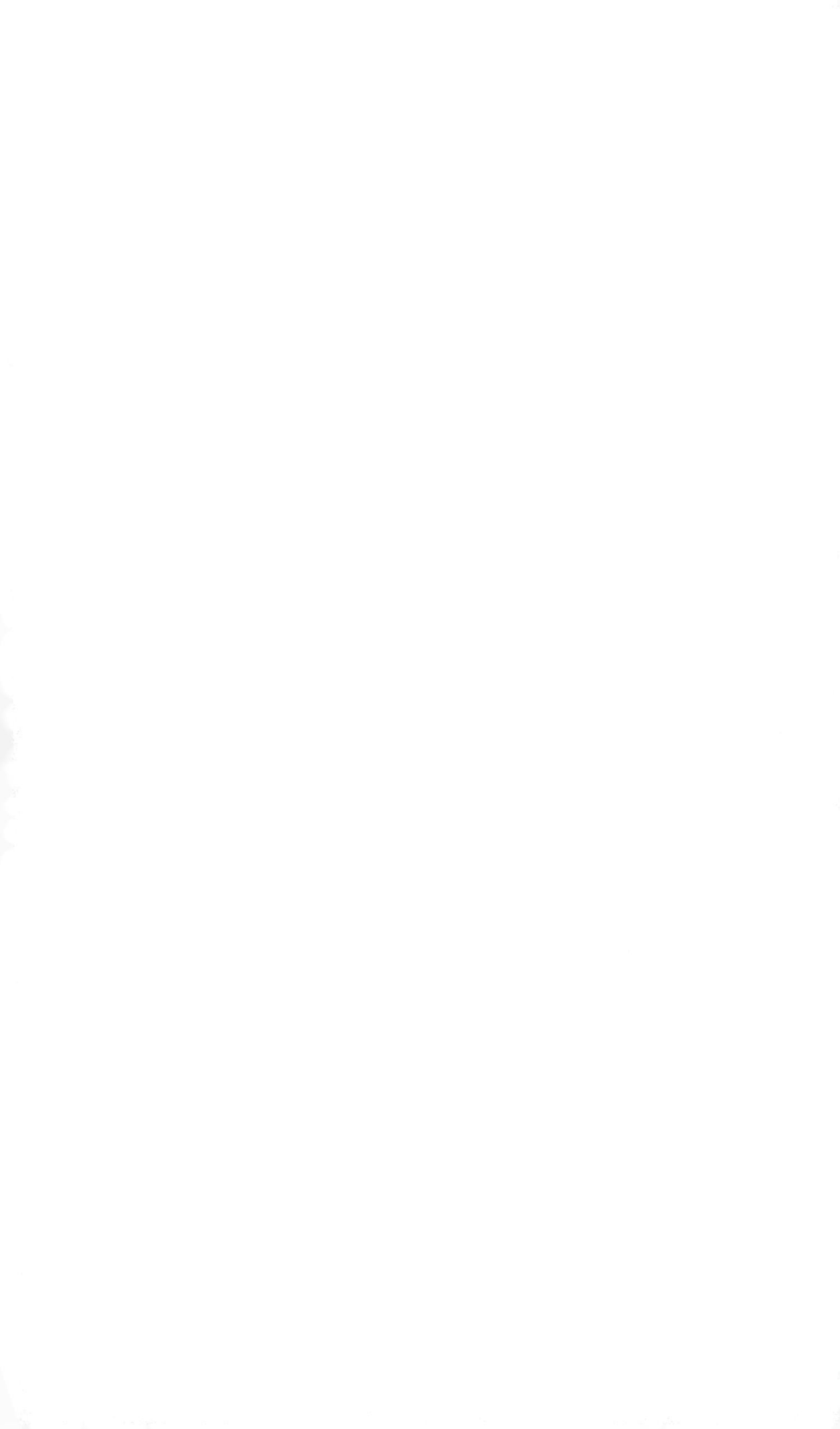